GUIDANCE FOR COVID-19

This book is a guide for the prevention and control measures issued by the Chinese Health Commission during the novel coronavirus pneumonia outbreak that has led to the global Covid-19 pandemic. With the guidance of this authoritative text, the number of cases in China has decreased from 83,386 to 2,000, and a complete victory in prevention and control will soon be achieved.

This book is suitable for professionals who are a part of the prevention and control of the plague, and for any readers who are concerned about their lives and the lives of their families and communities.

May God bless the world and bring us victory!

The National Health Commission (NHC) of the People's Republic of China is a cabinet-level executive department of the State Council which is responsible for formulating health policies in Mainland China. It was formed on 19 March 2018. The ministry is headquartered in Beijing. The commission is led by a Minister of cabinet rank in the state council.

www.royalcollins.com

GUIDANCE FOR
COVID-19

—

PREVENTION, CONTROL, DIAGNOSIS AND MANAGEMENT

Edited by
National Health Commission (NHC) of the PRC
National Administration of Traditional Chinese Medicine of the PRC

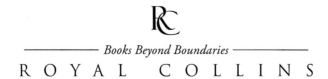

Books Beyond Boundaries

ROYAL COLLINS

Guidance for COVID-19: Prevention, Control, Diagnosis and Management

First published in 2020 by Royal Collins Publishing Group Inc.
Groupe Publication Royal Collins Inc.
BKM ROYALCOLLINS PUBLISHERS PRIVATE LIMITED

Headquarters: 550-555 boul. René-Lévesque O Montréal (Québec) H2Z1B1 Canada
India office: 805 Hemkunt House, 8th Floor, Rajendra Place, New Delhi 110 008

Original Edition © People's Medical Publishing House, 2020

Copyright © Royal Collins Publishing Group Inc.
Groupe Publication Royal Collins Inc.
BKM ROYALCOLLINS PUBLISHERS PRIVATE LIMITED

ISBN: 978-1-4878-0456-5 (paperback)
ISBN: 978-1-4878-0459-6 (ebook)

To find out more about our publications, please visit **www.royalcollins.com**

Preface

On December 29, 2019, a hospital in Wuhan, Hubei Province, China reported an outbreak of severe unexplained viral pneumonia. The Chinese government timely notified World Health Organization (WHO) about the outbreak after verification. On January 8, 2020, the pathogen of this outbreak was identified as the novel coronavirus 2019 (2019-nCoV), and its gene sequence was quickly submitted to WHO. On January 30, WHO declared the outbreak of the novel coronavirus pneumonia (NCP) as a public health emergency of international concern (PHEIC). On February 12, 2020, International Committee on Taxonomy of Viruses (ICTV) declared that 2019-nCoV was officially named as severe acute respiratory syndrome coronavirus 2 (SARS-CoV-2), and on the same day, WHO declared the disease caused by SARS-CoV-2 was officially named as corona virus disease 2019 (COVID-19).

The Chinese government gives top priority to the safety of people's life and health thus has taken the prevention and control of COVID-19 epidemic as the most important work at present. To control the COVID-19 outbreak, the National Health Commission of the People's Republic of China, along with the National Administration of Traditional Chinese Medicine and some other relative organizations, have organized experts to timely issue and update the guidelines for the COVID-19 diagnosis, treatment, prevention, and control. The guidelines were written based on the study, analysis and summary of the treatment of previous COVID-19 cases, and are used to guide medical staff and public health workers in China to better understand, prevent and treat the COVID-19.

In order to truthfully and objectively share China's COVID-19 diagnosis, treatment, prevention, and control experience with the world, we have translated the latest Chinese guidelines and their relevant interpretations in this book. We hope this book can provide references for other countries affected by the COVID-19, and also promote the experience exchange and cooperation in disease prevention, control, diagnosis and management, thus promote the development of global health together.

On behalf of the compilation and translation board of this book, we especially acknowledge Prof. Jinling TANG (from Guangzhou Women and Children's Medical Center) and Prof. Huaqing WANG (from Chinese Center for Disease Control and Prevention) for their help and support for the publication of this book.

Xiaofeng LIANG, Zijian FENG, and Liming LI

Compilation and Translation Board

Translators in Chief
Xiaofeng LIANG, Chinese Preventive Medicine Association, Beijing, China
Zijian FENG, Chinese Center for Disease Control and Prevention, Beijing, China
Liming LI, Peking University, Beijing, China

Committee Members
Zhenqiang BI, Shandong Center for Disease Control and Prevention, Jinan, China
Qingwu JIANG, Fudan University, Shanghai, China
Peng WANG, Chinese Preventive Medicine Association, Beijing, China
Yu JIANG, Peking Union Medical College & Chinese Academy of Medical
    Sciences, Beijing, China

Authors of Chapters of Development and Revisions of Plans/Guidelines
Rongmeng JIANG, Beijing Ditan Hospital, Capital Medical University, Beijing,
    China
Liping WANG, Chinese Center for Disease Control and Prevention, Beijing,
    China
Peng WANG, Chinese Preventive Medicine Association, Beijing, China

Translators
Yu JIANG, Yongle ZHAN, Yawen WANG, Mingyu SI, Jingwen ZHANG,
Mingshuang LI, Yunli CHEN, Yingjie SHI, Xuan LIU, Hexin YUE, Ao JING,
Tianchen LV, Yaohan MENG, Yimin QU, Yahui FENG, Baohu YAN, Sansan WU,
Shuya CAI, and Peng XUE

*School of Public Health, Peking Union Medical College & Chinese Academy of
Medical Sciences, Beijing, China*

Contents

Preface   *vi*

Compilation and Translation Board   *viii*

Part One   **Diagnosis and Treatment Plan of Corona Virus Disease 2019**   **1**

Chapter 1   Diagnosis and Treatment Plan of Corona Virus Disease 2019   3
(Tentative Sixth Edition)

Chapter 2   Interpretation of the Diagnosis and Treatment Plan of Corona Virus Disease 2019   17
(Tentative Fifth Revised Edition)

Chapter 3   Interpretation of the Diagnosis and Treatment Plan of Corona Virus Disease 2019   25
(Tentative Sixth Edition)

Chapter 4   Development and Revisions of the Diagnosis and Treatment Plan of Corona Virus Disease 2019   31
(Tentative First to Sixth Editions)

Part Two   **Prevention and Control Plan of Corona Virus Disease 2019**   **39**

Chapter 1   Prevention and Control Plan of Corona Virus Disease 2019   41
(Fourth Edition)

Chapter 2   Interpretation of the Prevention and Control Plan
of Corona Virus Disease 2019   91
(Fourth Edition)

Chapter 3   Development and Revisions of the Prevention
and Control Plan of Corona Virus Disease 2019   93
(First to Fourth Editions)

**Part Three   Guidelines for Prevention and Control
of 2019-nCoV**   **115**

Chapter 1   Guidelines for Prevention and Control
of 2019-nCoV   117
(First Edition)

Chapter 2   Interpretation of the Guidelines for Prevention
and Control of 2019-nCoV   131
(First Edition)

PART ONE

Diagnosis and Treatment Plan of Corona Virus Disease 2019

(Source: National Health Commission (NHC) of the PRC, General Office; National Administration of Traditional Chinese Medicine of the PRC, General Office)

Diagnosis and Treatment Plan of Corona Virus Disease 2019

(Tentative Sixth Edition)

Since December 2019, an increasing number of cases of novel coronavirus pneumonia (NCP) have been diagnosed in Wuhan, Hubei Province. With the spreading of the epidemic, cases (officially named as Corona Virus Disease 2019 [COVID-19] by WHO) have also been reported in other regions of China and abroad. COVID-19 was urgently classified, by the *Law of the People's Republic of China on the Prevention and Treatment of Infectious Diseases* as Class B communicable diseases, and is managed as Class A communicable diseases. With the in-depth understanding and accumulation of diagnosis and treatment experience of COVID-19, the *Diagnosis and Treatment Plan of Corona Virus Disease 2019* (the Tentative Fifth Revised Edition) was revised and formed the current tentative sixth edition.

1 Pathogenic Characteristics

The novel coronavirus 2019 (2019-nCoV, officially named as severe acute respiratory syndrome coronavirus 2 [SARS-CoV-2] by ICTV) belongs to the genus β, with envelope, round or elliptic and often pleomorphic form, and 60–140 nm in diameter. The virus genetically differs considerably from those of SARSr-CoV and MERSr-CoV. Current studies show that the homology between 2019-nCoV and bat-SARS-like coronavirus (bat-SL-CoVZC45) is over 85%. When cultured in vitro, 2019-nCoV can be found in human respiratory epithelial cells after about 96 hours, while it takes about 6 days to isolate and culture Vero E6 and Huh-7 cell lines.

Knowledge on the physical and chemical characteristics of coronaviruses is mainly derived from the study of SARSr-CoV and MERSr-CoV. Coronaviruses are sensitive to ultraviolet rays and heat, and can be effectively inactivated by heating at 56°C for 30 min and lipid solvents such as ether, 75% ethanol, chlorine-containing disinfectant, peroxyacetic acid and chloroform except chlorhexidine.

2 Epidemiological Characteristics

2.1 Source of Infection

At present, the major source of infection is the patients with COVID-19, and asymptomatic 2019-nCoV carriers seem also a potential source of infection.

2.2 Route of Transmission

COVID-19 is mainly transmitted by droplets and contact. Aerosol transmission is possible when people have prolonged exposure to high concentrations of aerosols in relatively closed spaces.

2.3 Susceptible Individuals

Humans of all ages are generally susceptible.

3 Clinical Characteristics

3.1 Clinical Manifestations

Based on current epidemiological investigations, the incubation period of COVID-19 is ranged between 1 to 14 days, and generally within 3 to 7 days.

Fever, fatigue and dry coughing are considered the main clinical manifestations, but symptoms such as stuffy nose, runny nose, pharyngalgia, myalgia and diarrhea are relatively less common. In severe cases, dyspnea and/or hypoxemia usually occurs after one week of disease onset, and the worse can rapidly progresses to acute respiratory distress syndrome, septic shock, metabolic acidosis hard to correct, and hemorrhage and coagulation dysfunction, multiple organ failure, etc. It's worth noting that patients with severe or critical illness may have a moderate to low fever, or no fever at all.

Mild cases only present with light fever, mild fatigue and so on without manifestation of pneumonia.

From the cases treated currently, most of the patients have a favorable prognosis. The elderly and people with chronic underlying diseases usually have poor prognosis while cases with relatively mild symptoms are common in children.

3.2 Laboratory Examination

In the early stage of COVID-19, a normal or decreased total white blood cell count and a decreased lymphocyte count can be found in patients. In addition, increased value of liver enzymes, LDH, muscle enzymes and myoglobin can occur in some patients; and raised level of troponin can be seen in some critically ill patients. In most cases, the laboratory tests show a raised C-reactive protein value and erythrocyte sedimentation rate but a normal procalcitonin value. Among severe patients, D-dimer value is increased and peripheral blood lymphocytes decreased persistently. In addition, elevated values of inflammatory factors are accompanied with in severe and critical patients.

The nucleic acid of 2019-nCoV can be detected in biological specimens such as nasopharyngeal swabs, sputum, other lower respiratory tract secretions, blood and feces.

To improve the positive rate of nucleic acid detection, it is recommended to collect and retain sputum in general patients besides those performed with tracheal intubation (lower respiratory tract secretions should be collected); and all the specimens should be sent and tested as fast as possible.

3.3 Chest Imaging

In the early stage of COVID-19, the images show that there are multiple small patched shadows and interstitial changes, especially in the lung periphery. As the disease progresses, the images of these patients further develop into multiple ground glass shadows and infiltration shadows in both lungs. In severe cases, lung consolidation may occur. It is seldom to find pleural effusion in patients with COVID-19.

4 Diagnostic Criteria

4.1 Suspected Cases

The suspected cases should be diagnosed through considering both the epidemiological histories and clinical manifestations:

4.1.1 Epidemiology

(1) Having a history of travel or residence in Wuhan and its surrounding areas or other communities with cases reported within 14 days before the patient's onset; or

(2) Having a contact history with patients (a positive results of nucleic acid test of 2019-nCoV) within 14 days before the patient's onset; or

(3) Having a contact history with patients with fever or respiratory symptoms from Wuhan and its surrounding areas, or the communities with cases reported within 14 days before the patient's onset; or

(4) Clustering occurrence of cases.

4.1.2 Clinical Manifestations

(1) Fever and/or respiratory symptoms;

(2) Having the imaging features of pneumonia described above;

(3) In the early stage, a normal or decreased total white blood cell count and a decreased lymphocyte count can be found.

Patients who satisfy any one of the epidemiological exposure histories as well as any two of the clinical manifestations can be diagnosed as suspected cases. Patients with no definite epidemiological history can be diagnosed only if all the three clinical manifestations are met.

4.2 Confirmed Cases

The suspected cases with one of the following etiological evidences can be diagnosed as confirmed cases:

(1) A positive result of the nucleic acid of 2019-nCoV by real-time fluorescence RT-PCR;

(2) The virus gene sequence is highly homologous to the known 2019-nCoV.

5 Clinical Classifications

5.1 Mild Cases

The clinical symptoms are mild and no pneumonia manifestation can be found in imaging.

5.2 Ordinary Cases

Patients have symptoms like fever and respiratory tract symptoms, etc. and pneumonia manifestation can be seen in imaging.

5.3 Severe Cases

Meeting any of the following:

(1) Respiratory distress, RR $\geq$ 30 breaths/min;

(2) Pulse oxygen saturation (SpO_2) $\leq$ 93% on room air at rest state;

(3) Arterial partial pressure of oxygen (PaO_2) / oxygen concentration (FiO_2) $\leq$ 300 mmHg (1 mmHg=0.133 kPa).

For high altitude areas (above 1 kilometer), PaO_2/FiO_2 values should be adjusted based on equation of $PaO_2/FiO_2 \times$ [Atmospheric Pressure (mmHg)/760].

Patients with >50% lesions progression within 24 to 48 hours in pulmonary imaging should be treated as severe cases.

5.4 Critical Cases

Meeting any of the following:

(1) Respiratory failure occurs and mechanical ventilation is required;

(2) Shock occurs;

(3) Complicated with other organ failure that requires monitoring and treatment in ICU.

6 Differential Diagnosis

6.1 The mild manifestations caused by COVID-19 should be distinguished from respiratory infections caused by other viruses.

6.2 NCP should be distinguished from viral pneumonia caused by influenza virus, adenovirus or respiratory syncytial virus, and mycoplasma pneumonia. Especially for suspected cases, rapid antigen detection, multiple PCR nucleic acid test and other methods should be adopted to examine common respiratory pathogens.

6.3 In addition, differentiation from non-infectious diseases such as vasculitis, dermatomyositis, and organizing pneumonia should also be performed.

7 Case Identification and Report

Medical staff at all levels and types of medical institutions should immediately isolate and treat every suspected case that meet the definition of the disease in a single room. After in-hospital experts' consultation or attending physicians' consultation, people still be considered as suspected cases need to be reported online within 2 hours. Specimens should be collected and tested for the nucleic acid of 2019-nCoV. Suspected patients should be transferred to the designated hospitals as soon as possible. People intimately contacted with COVID-19 patients or those even with positive results in common respiratory pathogens test, are also recommended to conduct the pathogenic detection 2019-nCoV in time.

8 Treatment

8.1 Determine the Treatment Place According to the Severity of the Disease

(1) Suspected and confirmed cases should be isolated and treated in designated hospitals with effective isolation and protective conditions. Suspected cases should be treated in single rooms, while confirmed cases can be admitted to the same ward.

(2) Critical cases should be admitted to ICU as soon as possible.

8.2 General Treatment

(1) Rest patients in bed, strengthen supportive treatment, and ensure adequate nutrition. Keep the balance of water and electrolyte to maintain the stability of the internal environment. Closely monitor vital signs, oxygen saturation, etc.

(2) Monitor blood routine, urine routine, CRP, biochemical indicators (liver enzyme, myocardial enzyme, renal function, etc.), coagulation function, arterial blood gas analysis, chest imaging, etc. according to the patient's condition. If possible, cytokine testing should be conducted.

(3) Give effective oxygen therapy measures in time, including nasal cannula, mask oxygen, high-flow nasal oxygen therapy.

(4) Antiviral Treatment: Give alpha-interferon nebulization (5 million units or equivalent per time for adult, add 2 mL of sterile water for injection, aerosol inhalation twice per day); lopinavir/ritonavir (200 mg/50 mg per capsule, 2 capsules each time, twice per day for adults, the course of treatment should be ≤10 days); ribavirin (combining with interferon or lopinavir/ritonavir are

recommended, 500 mg for adults per time, inject 2–3 times per day intra-venously, the course of treatment should be ≤10 days). Chloroquine phosphate (500 mg for adult, twice per day, the course of treatment should be ≤10 days), Arbidol (200 mg for adults, three times per day, the course of treatment should be ≤10 days). Keep alert on side effects such as diarrhea, nausea, vomiting, and liver damage related to lopinavir/ritonavir, as well as harmful interaction with other drugs. Effects of current trial drugs should be further evaluated during clinical usage. Simultaneously use of three or more types of antiviral drugs is not recommended and relevant drug treatment should stop if unbearable side effects occur.

(5) Antibacterial Drug Treatment: unselective or inappropriate use of antibiotics should be avoided, especially in combination with broad-spectrum antibiotics.

8.3 Treatment of Severe and Critical Cases

8.3.1 Treatment Principles

On the basis of symptomatic treatment, actively prevent complications, treat accompanying diseases, prevent secondary infections, and provide organ function support in time.

8.3.2 Respiratory Support

(1) Oxygen Therapy: Severe patients should be provided inhalation oxygen with facemask or nasal catheter. Timely assess whether respiratory distress and/or hypoxemia are relieved.

(2) High-Flow Nasal Catheter Oxygen Therapy or Non-Invasive Mechanical Ventilation: When respiratory distress and/or hypoxemia cannot be relieved after standard oxygen therapy, high-flow nasal catheter oxygen therapy or noninvasive ventilation should be considered. If the condition does not improve or even worsen within a short period of time (1–2 hours), endotracheal intubation and invasive mechanical ventilation should be performed promptly.

(3) Invasive Mechanical Ventilation: Use lung protective ventilation strategies, which means small tidal volume (4–8 mL/kg ideal weight) and low inspiratory pressure (platform pressure <30 cmH$_2$O) for mechanical ventilation to reduce ventilator-related lung injuries. For several patients, human-machine synchro-nization is not available, and sedative and muscle relaxants should be used in time.

(4) Salvage Treatment: For patients with severe ARDS, it is recommended to perform lung expansion. If possible, prone position ventilation should be

performed for more than 12 hours per day. For those with poor prone position ventilation, extracorporeal membrane oxygenation (ECMO) should be considered as soon as possible if conditions permit.

8.3.3 Circulation Support: On the basis of adequate fluid resuscitation, improve microcirculation, use vasoactive drugs, and perform hemodynamic monitoring when necessary.

8.3.4 Convalescent plasma therapy: suitable for treating rapidly developed cases, severe cases and critical cases. Administrations and dosage refer to *Clinical Plasma Therapy Plan for Corona Virus Disease 2019 Convalescents during Recovery (Tentative First Edition)*.

8.3.5 Other Treatments

According to the severity of respiratory distress and the progress of chest imaging, glucocorticoids can be used within a short period of time (3–5 days) as appropriate. Dose does not exceed the equivalent of 1–2 mg/kg/day of methylprednisolone is recommended. It should be noted that higher doses of glucocorticoids would delay coronavirus clearance due to immunosuppressive effects; Xuebijing Injection (a traditional Chinese medicine) can be given intravenously 100 mL/day, twice a day for treatment; microecological preparation can be used to keep the equilibrium for intestinal microecology and prevent secondary bacterial infection; Plasma exchange, adsorption, perfusion, blood/plasma filtering and other extracorporeal blood purification technologies should be considered if possible for critical cases with severe inflammatory reactions.

Anxiety and fear usually occur in many patients, therefore psychological counseling should be strengthened.

8.4 Traditional Chinese Medicine Treatment

COVID-19 can also be treated with traditional Chinese medicine, which considers it caused by epidemic pathogenic factors located in the lungs. Different regions can refer to the following schemes for dialectical treatment according to the disease condition, local climate characteristics, and different physical conditions. Use drugs under the guidance of doctors if the dose of drug exceeds the pharmacopoeia.

8.4.1 Medical Observation Period

Clinical Manifestation 1: fatigue with gastrointestinal upset

Recommended Chinese Medicine: Huoxiangzhengqi Capsule (pill, oral liquid)

Clinical Manifestation 2: fatigue with fever

Recommended Chinese Medicines: Jinhua Qinggan Granules, Lianhua Qingwen Capsules (granules), Shufeng Jiedu Capsules (granules).

8.4.2 Clinical Treatment Period (For Confirmed Cases)

(1) Lung-Clearing and Detoxification Soup

Application Scope: suitable for mild, general and severe cases; reasonable for treating critical cases according to clinical symptoms.

Basic Prescription: *Herba Ephedrae* 9 g, roasted *Radix Glycyrrhizae* 6 g, *Semen Armeniacae Amarum* 9 g, raw *Gypsum Fibrosum* 15–30 g (decocted first), *Ramulus Cinnamomi* 9 g, *Rhizoma Alismatis* 9 g, *Polyporus Umbellatus* 9 g, *Rhizoma Atractylodis Macrocephalae* 9 g, *Poria* 15 g, *Radix Bupleuri* 16 g, *Radix Scutellariae* 6 g, *Rhizoma Pinelliae Preparata* 9 g, *Rhizoma Zingiberis Recens* 9 g, *Radix Asteris* 9 g, *Flos Farfarae* 9 g, *Rhizoma Belamcandae* 9 g, *Herba Asari* 6 g, *Rhizoma Dioscoreae* 12 g, *Fructus Aurantii Immaturus* 6 g, *Pericarpium Citri Reticulatae* 6 g, *Herba Pogostemonis* 9 g.

Administrations and Dosage: The basic prescription is a traditional Chinese medicine, which should be decocted by water for drink. Decoct same drugs twice per day, in the morning and in the evening (40 minutes after meals), three pieces are regarded as a course of treatment.

Take half bowl of rice soup if possible after taking the medicine, or a bowl of rice soup for people with dry tongue and deficient body fluid. (Notes: the dosage of raw gypsum should be decreased for people without fever, and be increased for people with mild or severe fever.) Take the second course of treatment if the symptoms are improve but not disappeared, and it can be modified according to the actual situation for people with special requirements or other basic diseases. The medicine should be discontinued if the symptoms disappear.

Sources of Prescription: *Recommendation of Lung-Clearing and Detoxification Soup in the Treatment of Corona Virus Disease 2019 by Integrated Traditional Chinese and Western Medicine* (No. (2020)22, the Ministry of Traditional Chinese Medicine) issued by the Office of National Health Commission and Office of National Administration of Traditional Chinese Medicine.

(2) Mild Type

1) Cold Dampness Stagnating Lungs

Clinical Manifestations: fever, fatigue, soreness, coughing, expectoration, chest tightness, suffocation, nausea, vomiting and sticky stools. Pale or red tongue with fat tooth marks, moss white thick rotten or greasy fur, and soft and floating or slippery pulse.

Recommended Prescription: Raw *Herba Ephedrae* 6 g, raw *Gypsum Fibrosum* 15 g, *Semen Armeniacae Amarum* 9 g, *Rhizoma et Radix Notopterygii* 15 g, *Semen Lepidii* 15 g, *Rhizoma Cyrtomii* 9 g, *Lumbricus* 15 g, *Radix Cynanchi Paniculati* 15 g, *Herba Pogostemonis* 15 g, *Herba Eupatorii* 9 g, *Rhizoma Atractylodis* 15 g, *Poria* 45 g, raw *Rhizoma Atractylodis Macrocephalae* 30 g, charred *Fructus Hordei Germinatus*, charred *Fructus Crataegi* and charred *Massa Medicata Fermentata* 9 g each, *Cortex Magnoliae Officinalis* 15 g, charred *Semen Arecae* 9 g, *Fructus Tsaoko* 9 g, *Rhizoma Zingiberis Recens* 15 g.

Administrations and Dosage: One dose per day, decocted with 600 mL water, taken in the morning, noon and evening respectively before meals.

2) Damp-Heat Accumulated Lung

Clinical Manifestations: low fever or normal body temperature, slight chills alternate, head and body heaviness, muscle soreness, dry cough and less sputum, sore throat, dry mouth and no desire to drink, or chest tightness, epigastric fullness, no sweat or unsmooth sweating, or vomiting, nausea, loose stool or constipation. Pale or red tongue with white, thick, greasy or thin yellow fur, and smooth or moist pulse.

Recommended Prescription: *Semen Arecae* 10 g, *Fructus Tsaoko* 10 g, *Cortex Magnoliae Officinalis* 10 g, *Rhizoma Anemarrhenae* 10 g, *Radix Scutellariae* 10 g, *Radix Bupleuri* 10 g, *Radix Paeoniae Rubra* 10 g, *Fructus Forsythiae* 15 g, *Herba Artemisiae Annuae* 10 g (decocted later), *Rhizoma Atractylodis* 10 g, *Folium Isatidis* 10 g, raw *Radix Glycyrrhizae* 5 g.

Administrations and Dosage: One dose per day, decocted with 400 mL water, taken once in the morning and once in the evening.

(3) General Type

1) Damp-Poison Stagnating Lung

Clinical Manifestations: fever, cough with less sputum or yellow sputum, chest tightness, shortness of breath, abdominal distension. Dark red and fat tongue with yellow greasy or dry fur, rapid and/or slippery pulses.

Recommended Prescription: raw *Herba Ephedrae* 6 g, *Semen Armeniacae Amarum* 15 g, raw *Gypsum Fibrosum* 30 g, raw *Semen Coicis* 30 g, *Rhizoma Atractylodis* 10 g, *Herba Pogostemonis* 15 g, *Herba Artemisiae Annuae* 12 g,

Rhizoma Polygoni Cuspidati 20 g, *Herba Verbenae* 30 g, Dry *Rhizoma Phragmitis* 30 g, *Semen Lepidii* 15 g, *Exocarpium Citri Grandis* 15 g, *Radix Glycyrrhizae* 10 g.

Administrations and Dosage: one dose per day, decocted with 400 ml water, taken once in the morning and once in the evening.

2) Cold Dampness Obstructing Lung

Clinical Manifestations: Low fever, hiding fever, or no fever, dry cough, little sputum, fatigue, chest tightness, nausea, or vomiting, loose stools. Pale or red tongue, white greasy fur, soft and floating pulse.

Recommended Prescription: *Rhizoma Atractylodis* 15 g, *Pericarpium Citri Reticulatae* 10 g, *Cortex Magnoliae Officinalis* 10 g, *Herba Pogostemonis* 10 g, *Fructus Tsaoko* 6 g, raw *Herba Ephedrae* 6 g, *Rhizoma et Radix Notopterygii* 10 g, *Rhizoma Zingiberis Recens* 10 g, *Semen Arecae* 10 g.

Administrations and Dosage: One dose per day, decocted with 400 mL water, taken once in the morning and once in the evening.

(4) Severe Type

1) Lung Blocked by Epidemic Toxin

Clinical Manifestations: fever, flushing, cough, less yellow sticky sputum with or without blood, wheezing and shortness of breath, fatigue, bitter and sticky dry mouth, nausea with anorexia, poor stool movements, less brown urine. Red tongue with yellow greasy, slippery pulse.

Recommended Prescription: Raw *Herba Ephedrae* 6 g, *Semen Armeniacae Amarum* 9 g, *Gypsum Fibrosum* 15 g, *Radix Glycyrrhizae* 3 g, *Herba Pogostemonis* 10 g (decocted later), *Cortex Magnoliae Officinalis* 10 g, *Rhizoma Atractylodis* 15 g, *Fructus Tsaoko* 10 g, *Rhizoma Pinelliae Preparatum* 9 g, *Poria* 15 g, raw *Radix et Rhizoma Rhei* 5 g (decocted later), raw *Radix Astragali seu Hedysari* 10 g, *Semen Lepidii* 10 g, *Radix Paeoniae Rubra* 10 g.

Administrations and Dosage: One or two doses per day, decocted with 100–200 mL water, taken 2–4 times a day, oral or nasal feeding.

2) Flaring Heat in Qi and Ying

Clinical Manifestations: severe fever and polydipsia, dyspnea and anhelation, delirium, blurred vision, rash, or hematemesis and epistaxis, or convulsion of the limbs. Tongue with little or no fur, deep and count pulse, or large and rapid pulse.

Recommended Prescription: Raw *Gypsum Fibrosum* 30–60 g (decocted first), *Rhizoma Anemarrhenae* 30 g, *Radix Rehmanniae* 30–60 g, *Cornu Bubali* 30 g (decocted first), *Radix Paeoniae Rubra* 30 g, *Radix Scrophulariae* 30 g, *Fructus Forsythiae* 15 g, *Cortex Moutan* 15 g, *Rhizoma Coptidis* 6 g, *Folium Phyllostachydis Henonis* 12 g, *Semen Lepidii* 15 g, *Radix Glycyrrhizae* 6 g.

Administrations and Dosage: One dose per day, decocted with 100 mL to 200 mL water, decoct Gypsum Fibrosum and Cornu Bubali firstly, taken 2 to 4 times per day, oral or nasal feeding.

Recommend Chinese Medicine: Xiyanping injection, Xuebijing injection, Reduning injection, Tanreqing injection, Xingnaojing injection. Drugs with similar effects may be selected according to individual conditions or may be used jointly according to clinical symptoms. Traditional Chinese medicine injection can be used in combination with decoction.

(5) Critical Type (Internal Block and Outward Desertion)
Clinical Manifestations: dyspnea, asthma requires assisted ventilation, dizziness, irritability, cold sweaty limbs, purple tongue, thick or dry fur, large floating and rootless pulse.

Recommended Prescription: *Radix Ginseng* 15 g, *Radix Aconiti Lateralis Preparata* 10 g (decocted first), *Fructus Corni* 15 g, drinking with Suhexiang Pills or Angong Niuhuang Pills.

Recommended Chinese Medicine: Xuebijing Injection, Reduning Injection, Tanreqing Injection, Xingnaojing Injection, Shenfu Injection, Shengmai Injection 1, Shengmai Injection 2. Drugs with similar effects may be selected according to individual conditions or may be used jointly according to clinical symptoms. Traditional Chinese medicine injection can be used in combination with decoction.

Notes: Recommended Usage of Traditional Chinese Medicine Injections for Severe and Critical Cases

The use of traditional Chinese medicine injections should follow the principle of starting with low dose and modifying gradually and dialectically according to the drug instructions. The recommended usage is as follows:

Viral Infection or Combined with Mild Bacterial Infection: 0.9% Sodium Chloride Injection 250 mL and Xiyanping Injection 100 mg bid, or 0.9% Sodium Chloride Injection 250 mL and Reduning Injection 20 mL, or 0.9% Sodium Chloride Injection 250 mL and Tanreqing Injection 40 mg bid.

Severe Fever with Consciousness Disturbance: Xingnao Injection 20 mL and 0.9% Sodium Chloride Injection 250 mL, bid, twice daily.

Systemic Inflammatory Response Syndrome (SIRS) and/or multiple organ failure: Xuebijing Injection 100 mL and 0.9% Sodium Chloride Injection 250 mL, bid, twice daily.

Immunosuppression: Shengmai Injection 100 mL and 0.9% Sodium Chloride Injection 250 mL, bid, twice daily.

Shock: Shenfu Injection 100 mL and 0.9% Sodium Chloride Injection 250 mL, bid, twice daily.

(6) Recovery Period

1) Lung Deficiency and Spleen Qi

Clinical Manifestations: shortness of breath, tiredness, anorexia, distention and fullness, constipation, loose stool, pale tongue, whitish greasy fur.

Recommended Prescription: *Rhizoma Pinelliae Preparatum* 9 g, *Pericarpium Citri Reticulatae* 10 g, *Radix Codonopsis* 15 g, roasted *Radix Astragali seu Hedysari* 30 g, roasted *Rhizoma Atractylodis Macrocephalae* 10 g, *Poria* 15 g, *Herba Pogostemonis* 10 g, *Fructus Amomi Villosi* 6 g (decocted later), *Radix Glycyrrhizae* 6 g.

Administrations and Dosage: One dose per day, decocted with 400 mL water, take once in the morning and once in the evening.

2) Deficiency of Qi and Yin

Clinical Manifestations: fatigue, shortness of breath, dry mouth, thirst, hyperhidrosis, anorexia, low fever or no fever, dry cough, less sputum, dry tongue, thin or weak pulse.

Recommended Prescription: *Radix Adenophorae* 10 g, *Radix Glehniae* 10 g, *Radix Ophiopogonis* 15 g, *Radix Panacis Quinquefolii* 6 g, *Fructus Schisandrae Chinensis* 6 g, raw *Gypsum Fibrosum* 15 g, *Herba Lophatheri* 10 g, *Folium Mori* 10 g, *Rhizoma Phragmitis* 15 g, *Radix Salviae Miltiorrhizae* 15 g, *Radix Glycyrrhizae* 6 g.

Administrations and Dosage: One dose per day, decocted with 400 mL water, intake once in the morning and once in the evening.

9 Release of Isolation and Notes after Discharge

9.1 Release of Isolation and Discharge Standards

(1) With normal body temperature for more than 3 days;
(2) With significantly recovered respiratory symptoms;
(3) Lung imaging shows obvious absorption and recovery of acute exudative lesion;

(4) With negative results of the nucleic acid tests of respiratory pathogens for consecutive two times (sampling interval at least 1 day).

Patients meeting the standards mentioned above can be released from the isolation and discharged.

9.2 Notes after Discharge

(1) Designated hospitals should strengthen communication with basic medical institutions in patients' residence, share medical records, and forward information of discharged cases to relevant neighborhood committee and basic medical institutions.

(2) Discharged cases are recommended for continuous health monitor for 14 days, wearing facial masks, living in a ventilated single room, reducing frequency of close contact with family members, eating alone, keeping hand hygiene and avoiding outdoor activities due to the compromised immunome and risk of being infected with other pathogens.

(3) A follow-up and return visit in the second and fourth weeks respectively after discharge is recommended.

10 Transfer Principle

In accordance with the *Novel Coronavirus Pneumonia Case Transfer Program* (Tentative Edition) issued by our Commission.

11 Hospital Infection Control

Strictly comply with the requirements of the *Technical Guide for the Prevention and Control of Novel Coronavirus Infection in Medical Institutions* (First Edition) and *Guidelines for Usage of Common Medical Protective Equipment in Protection of Novel Coronavirus Pneumonia* (Tentative Edition).

CHAPTER 2

Interpretation of the Diagnosis and Treatment Plan of Corona Virus Disease 2019

(Tentative Fifth Revised Edition)*

On February 8th, 2020, National Health Commission of the People's Republic of China issued the *Diagnosis and Treatment Plan of Corona Virus Disease 2019* (Tentative Fifth Revised Edition).

Since December 2019, Wuhan City, Hubei Province has successively discovered multiple cases of patients with COVID-19. With the spread of the epidemic, other cases in China and abroad have also been found. Most of the currently reported cases have a history of residence or travel in Wuhan, but cases without that have already been found in some areas. As an acute respiratory infectious disease, COVID-19 has been classified into the Class B communicable diseases stipulated by the Law of the People's Republic of China on the Prevention and Treatment of Infectious Diseases, and managed as a Class A communicable diseases.

After the outbreak, National Health Commission organized relevant experts to formulate the tentative first edition, second edition, third edition, fourth edition and fifth edition of *Diagnosis and Treatment Plan of Corona Virus Disease 2019*.

The tentative fifth revised edition includes the characteristics of coronavirus pathogens, clinical characteristics, case definitions, differential diagnosis, case identify and report, treatment, release of isolation and discharge standards, transfer principles, and nosocomial infection control.

---

* In order to better understand the revised content from the tentative fifth revised edition to the tentative sixth edition of the *Diagnosis and Treatment Plan of Corona Virus Disease 2019*, this part adds the interpretation of the *Diagnosis and Treatment Plan of Corona Virus Disease 2019* (Tentative Fifth Revised Edition).

1 Characteristics of Coronavirus Pathogens

The coronavirus subfamilies are categorized into four genera: α, β, γ, and δ. Coupled with this newly discovered coronavirus, seven types of coronaviruses are known to infect humans. Most coronaviruses cause upper respiratory tract infections, but Middle East respiratory syndrome coronavirus (MERSr-CoV), severe acute respiratory syndrome associated coronavirus (SARSr-CoV) and novel coronavirus 2019 (2019-nCoV) can cause mild and even severe pneumonia, and can be transmitted from person to person.

Coronaviruses are sensitive to ultraviolet rays and heat, and can be effectively inactivated by a majority of disinfectants except chlorhexidine. Therefore, hand sanitizers containing chlorhexidine are not recommended for use here.

2 Epidemiological Characteristics

The source of infection is changed to *"The major source of infection currently is the patients with COVID-19, and asymptomatic 2019-nCoV carriers can also be the source of infection"*.

3 Clinical Characteristics

The incubation period of COVID-19 is 1 to 14 days, and generally within 3 to 7 days. Fever, fatigue and dry cough are considered the main manifestations along with symptoms such as stuffy nose, runny nose, and diarrhea in a few patients. Because some severe patients have no obvious dyspnea and present with hypoxemia, the text is changed to *"In severe cases, dyspnea and/or hypoxemia usually occurs after a week of disease onset, and the worse can rapidly progress to acute respiratory distress syndrome, septic shock, metabolic acidosis that is hard to balance, and hemorrhage and coagulation dysfunction, etc.".* This edition highlights that *"Mild patients only present with low fever, mild fatigue and so on, but without manifestation of pneumonia"*.

In terms of laboratory examination, this edition adds the following descriptions, "Increased values of liver enzymes, LDH, muscle enzymes and myoglobin can occur in some patients; and raised level of troponin can be seen in some critical patients" and "The nucleic acid of 2019-nCoV can be detected in biological specimens such asnasopharyngeal swabs, sputum, secretions of lower respiratory tract, blood and feces".

In the early stage of COVID-19, the images show that there are multiple small patches shadows and interstitial changes, especially in the lung periphery. As the disease progresses, the images of these patients further develop into multiple ground glass shadows and infiltration shadows in both lungs. In severe cases, lung consolidation may occur. It is seldom to find pleural effusion in patients with COVID-19.

4 Case Diagnosis

It is different between Hubei Province and other provinces.

Cases in other provinces except Hubei are still classified into "suspected cases" and "confirmed cases". Based on the fact that confirmed cases with no definite epidemiological exposure history have been found, "Those without definite epidemiological exposure history but meeting the three clinical manifestations (fever and/or respiratory symptoms; having the imaging features of pneumonia mentioned above; in the early stage, a normal or decrease of total white blood cells count and a decrease of lymphocyte count can be found)" are also included in the investigation of suspected cases. The diagnostic criteria for confirmed cases remain unchanged. (A positive result of the nucleic acid of 2019-nCoV by real-time fluorescence RT-PCR in respiratory tract specimens or blood specimens, or the virus gene sequence of respiratory tract specimens or blood specimens is highly homologous to the known 2019-nCoV.)

A classification of *"clinical diagnosis cases"* was added in Hubei Province. Moreover, the standard of "suspected cases" is revised to, *"Patients regardless of whether with an epidemiological history can be considered suspected cases as long as they satisfy the two clinical manifestations: 'fever and/or respiratory symptoms' and 'in the early stage, a normal or decrease of total white blood cells count and a decrease of lymphocyte count can be found'"*. It means that the diagnostic criteria of suspected cases has been relaxed. Suspected cases with imaging features of pneumonia are clinically diagnosed cases. The diagnostic criteria for confirmed cases remain unchanged.

5 Clinical Classifications

According to whether with clinical symptoms or pneumonia, the severity of pneumonia, whether with respiratory failure or shock, and whether with other organs failure, cases are divided into mild cases (clinical symptoms are mild, and no pneumonia can be found in imaging); ordinary cases (with symptoms like fever and respiratory tract, etc. and pneumonia manifestation can be seen in imaging); severe cases (respiratory distress, RR ≥ 30 breaths/min; pulse oxygen saturation (SpO_2) ≤ 93% on room air at rest state; arterial partial pressure of oxygen (PaO_2)/ oxygen concentration (FiO_2) ≤ 300 mmHg); and critical cases (respiratory failure occurs and mechanical ventilation is required; shock occurs; complicated with other organ failure that requires monitoring and treatment in ICU).

6 Differential Diagnosis

There are more than 100 species of pathogens that cause community-acquired pneumonia, of which viruses account for about 30%, and others viruses which cause pneumonia have something in common with the common influenza virus, parainfluenza virus, adenovirus, respiratory syncytial virus, rhinovirus, human metapneumovirus, SARS-CoV, etc. It is difficult to distinguish from clinical manifestations and chest imaging alone, while pathogenic testing is needed.

7 Case Identification, Report and Exclusion

Hubei Province is different from other provinces.

In provinces other than Hubei, the case identification and reporting procedures are same as the fourth edition of the Diagnosis and Treatment Plan, but the present edition emphasizes the safety of transfer and transfer the suspected patient to the designated hospital as soon as possible.

For Hubei Province, medical staff at all levels and types of medical institutions are required to immediately isolate and treat suspected and clinically diagnosed cases that meet the definition of the case. Every suspected or clinically diagnosed case should be isolated in a single room. And the specimens should be collected for pathogenic testing as soon as possible.

Suspected cases can be excluded after the nucleic acid test for respiratory pathogens is negative for two consecutive times (sampling interval at least 1 day).

8 Treatment

The treatments include isolation, symptomatic support, and close monitoring of condition changes, especially breathing rate and finger pulse oxygen saturation.

Every suspected case should be treated in single room, while confirmed cases can be admitted to the same ward.

Critical cases should be admitted to the ICU as soon as possible.

Antibiotics use: blind or inappropriate use of antibiotics should be avoided, especially in combination with broad-spectrum antibiotics.

Antiviral treatment: this edition adds the description of "no effective antiviral treatment is currently confirmed". Based on trying drugs of alpha-interferon aerosol inhalation and lopinavir/ritonavir, "or add ribavirin" is supplemented. After full discussion by the National COVID-19 Medical Treatment Expert Group, the dosage of ribavirin has been adjusted to 500 mg each time for adults with 2 to 3 times of intravenous infusions per day, considering the safety of its high-dose. At the same time, pay attention to lopinavir/ritonavir associated side effects, such as diarrhea, nausea, vomiting, liver damage, and the interactions with other drugs.

The key to reduce case fatality rate is successful treatment of severe and critical cases. Prevent and cure complications actively, treat basic diseases, prevent secondary infections, and provide timely organ function supports. Patients always feel anxious and frightened, psychological counseling should be strengthened.

On monitoring of disease, "cytokine detection is feasible for those people who have condition" has been supplemented.

Respiratory support: (1) Oxygen therapy: severe patients should be provided inhalation oxygen with facemask or nasal catheter, and timely assess whether respiratory distress and/or hypoxemia are relieved. (2) High-flow nasal catheter oxygen therapy or non-invasive mechanical ventilation: when respiratory distress and/or hypoxemia cannot be relieved after standard oxygen therapy, high-flow nasal catheter oxygen therapy or noninvasive ventilation should be considered. It is highlighted that "*if the condition does not improve or even worsen within a short time (1–2 hours), endotracheal intubation and invasive mechanical ventilation should be performed promptly*". (3) Invasive mechanical ventilation: lung protective ventilation strategies should be used, which means small tidal volume (4–8 ml/kg ideal weight) and low inspiratory pressure (platform pressure < 30 cmH$_2$O) for mechanical ventilation to reduce ventilator-related lungs injuries. (4) For patients with severe ARDS, it is recommended to perform lung expansion. If possible, prone position ventilation should be performed for more than 12 hours per day. For those with poor prone position ventilation, extracorporeal membrane oxygenation (ECMO) should be considered as soon as possible if conditions permit.

Circulation support: on the basis of adequate fluid resuscitation, improve microcirculation, use vasoactive drugs, and perform hemodynamic monitoring when necessary.

Other treatment measures: Glucocorticoids can be used in a short period of time (3–5 days) according to the severity of respiratory distress and the progress of chest imaging. The recommended dose of methylprednisolone should not exceed 1–2 mg/kg/day. It should be noted that higher doses of glucocorticoids would delay coronavirus clearance due to immunosuppressive effects. Xuebijing Injection (a traditional Chinese medicine) can be given intravenously 100 mL/day, twice a day for treatment. Microecological preparation can be used to keep the equilibrium for intestinal microecology and prevent secondary bacterial infection. Convalescent plasma therapy can be used. For critically ill patients with high inflammatory response, extracorporeal blood purification technology can be considered when conditions permit.

Chinese medicine treatment measures: COVID-19 belongs to the category of traditional Chinese medicine epidemic disease. It is caused by the epidemic pathogenic factors, and is located in the lung. The basic pathogenesis of COVID-19 is characterized by dampness, heat, poison, and silt. Different regions can refer to the following schemes for dialectical treatment according to the disease condition, local climate characteristics, and different physical conditions.

9 Release of Isolation and Discharge Standards

Based on "with normal body temperature for more than 3 days, and significantly recovered respiratory symptoms", that *"with obvious features of absorption of inflammation shown in lung imaging"* has been added. In addition, patients should also meet the criterion of negative results of the nucleic acid tests of respiratory pathogens for consecutive two times (sampling interval at least 1 day). Only all the above criteria satisfying can the patients be released from the hospital or transferred to the corresponding departments for other diseases according to their conditions.

10 Transfer Principle

In order to ensure the safety of transport, patients should be transported in special vehicles, personal protection of transport personnel and vehicle disinfection should be done.

CHAPTER 3

Interpretation of the Diagnosis and Treatment Plan of Corona Virus Disease 2019

(Tentative Sixth Edition)

On February 19th, 2020, National Health Commission of the People's Republic of China issued the *Diagnosis and Treatment Plan of Corona Virus Disease 2019* (Tentative Sixth Edition). And now, it is interpreted as follow.

1 Route of Transmission

"COVID-19 is mainly transmitted by respiratory droplets and contact" is changed to *"COVID-19 is mainly transmitted by respiratory droplets and close contact"*, in other words, "close" has been added in front of "contact". Besides, *"Aerosol transmission is possible when humans have prolonged exposure to high concentrations of aerosol in a relatively closed space"* is added.

2 Clinical Characteristics

In severe cases, in addition to *"rapidly progressing to acute respiratory distress syndrome, septic shock, difficult to correct metabolic acidosis, and hemorrhage and coagulation dysfunction"*, *"multiple organ failure"* can also occur in the worse.

As for laboratory examination, it is emphasized that *"To improve the positive rate of nucleic acid detection, it is recommended to collect and retain sputum in general patients except those performed with tracheal intubation (lower respiratory tract secretions should be collect); and all the specimens should be sent and tested as fast as possible."*

3 Case Diagnosis

Differences of diagnosis criteria between Hubei Province and other provinces were deleted and unified as "*suspected cases*" and "*confirmed cases*".

There are two judgements of suspected cases. First, "patients meet any one of the epidemiological exposure histories as well as any two of the clinical manifestations *(fever and/or respiratory symptoms; having the imaging features of pneumonia mentioned above; in the early stage, a normal or decrease of total white blood cells count and a decrease of lymphocyte count can be found)*. Second," *patients without definite epidemiological exposure history but meet the three clinical manifestations (fever and/or respiratory symptoms; having the imaging features of pneumonia mentioned above; in the early stage, a normal or decrease of total white blood cells count and a decrease of lymphocyte count can be found)*".

Positive pathogen evidences are required for confirmed cases (a positive result of the nucleic acid of 2019-nCoV by real-time fluorescence RT-PCR, or the virus gene sequence is highly homologous to the known 2019-nCoV).

4 Clinical Classifications

Cases are still divided into mild cases, ordinary cases, severe cases and critical cases. "*For high altitude areas (above 1 kilometer), PaO_2/FiO_2 values should be adjusted based on equation of $PaO_2/FiO_2 \times$ [Atmospheric Pressure (mmHg)/760]*" is added in the description of arterial partial pressure of oxygen (PaO_2)/ oxygen concentration (FiO_2) ≤ 300 mmHg.

Patients with "*>50% lesions progression within 24 to 48 hours in pulmonary imaging*" should be treated as severe cases.

5 Differential Diagnosis

Differential diagnosis should be performed according to mild cases of COVID-19 and NCP.

For example, the mild manifestations caused by COVID-19 should be distinguished from respiratory infections caused by other viruses. NCP should be distinguished from viral pneumonia caused by influenza virus, adenovirus or respiratory syncytial virus, and mycoplasma pneumonia.

"*Especially for suspected cases, rapid antigen detection, multiple PCR nucleic acid test and other methods should be adopted to examine common respiratory pathogens."* are highlighted in this edition.

6 Case Identification and Report

The *"Disposal requirements for clinical diagnosed case in Hubei Province"* is deleted.

In addition, *"Exclusion Criteria for Suspected Cases"* is also deleted. Standards of release of isolation for suspected cases are corresponded with *"Removal Standards of Isolation of Confirmed Case"*.

7 Treatment

(1) Determine the treatment place according to the severity of the disease. The *"Suspected cases and confirmed cases"* is deleted and *"Cases should be isolated and treated in designated hospitals with effective isolation and protective conditions. Confirmed cases can be admitted to the same ward."* is added.

(2) Antiviral treatment. The description of *"no effective antiviral treatment is currently confirmed"* is deleted. *"Chloroquine phosphate (500 mg for adult, twice per day)"* and *"Arbidol (200 mg for adult, three times per day)"* are added as trial drugs. Combinations of ribavirin and interferon or lopinavir/ritonavir are recommended. The course of treatment with trial drugs should be ≤10 days. Effects of trial drugs are recommended to be evaluated during clinical usage. Simultaneously use of three or more types of antiviral drugs is not recommended and relative drug treatment should stop if unbearable side effects occur.

(3) As for treatment to severe and critical cases, "convalescent plasma therapy" is added and recommended for treating rapidly developed cases, severe cases and critical cases. Administrations and dosage refer to *Clinical Plasma Therapy Plan for Corona Virus Disease 2019 Convalescents during Recovery* (Tentative First Edition).

(4) Other treatments. *"Extracorporeal blood purification technology should be considered if possible"* is changed to *"Plasma change, adsorption, perfusion, blood/ plasma filtering and other extracorporeal blood purification technologies should be considered if possible"* for critical cases with severe inflammatory reactions.

(5) Chinese medicine treatment. The *Diagnosis and Treatment Plan of Corona Virus Disease 2019* (Tentative Fifth Revised Edition) is modified and comple-

mented based on the in-depth observation and treatment of cases, summary and analysis of national-wide prescriptions of traditional Chinese medicine, screening effective experiences and prescriptions, and announcement of the *Recommendation of Lung-Clearing and Detoxification Soup in the Treatment of Corona Virus Disease 2019 by Integrated Traditional Chinese and Western Medicine*, the *Diagnosis and Treatment Plan of Severe and Critical Corona Virus Disease 2019 Cases* (Tentative Second Edition), and the *Management Regulation of Mild and General Corona Virus Disease 2019 Cases*. The classifications of stages of disease are consistent with the fifth revised edition and the traditional Chinese medicine treatment is divided into medical observation period and clinical treatment period (for confirmed cases), which is further divided into mild, general, severe, critical and recovery periods. Chinese patent medicine is recommended for medical observation period therapy while commonly used prescription, lung-clearing and detoxification soup is recommended for clinical treatment period. Interpretations of clinical manifestations, recommended prescription and dosage and intake methods are provided separately for mild, general, severe, critical and recovery periods. The specific usages of Chinese patent medicine (including traditional Chinese medicine injection) for severe and critical cases are added in the meantime. Different regions can refer to the recommended prescriptions for dialectical treatment according to the disease conditions, local climate characteristics, and different physical conditions.

8 Release of Isolation and Notes after Discharge

8.1 Release of isolation should meet with the following four standards:

(1) Having normal body temperature for more than 3 days;

(2) With significantly recovered respiratory symptoms;

(3) Lung imaging shows obvious absorption and recovery of acute exudative lesion;

(4) With negative results of the nucleic acid tests of respiratory pathogens for consecutive twice (sampling interval at least 1 day).

8.2 *"Notes after discharge"* is added:

(1) Designated hospitals should strengthen communication with basic medical

institutions in patients' residence, share medical records, and forward information of discharged cases to relevant neighborhood committee and basic medical institutions.

(2) Discharged cases are recommended for continuously health monitor for 14 days, wearing facial masks, living in a ventilated single room, reducing frequency of close contact with family members, eating alone, keeping hand hygiene and avoiding outdoor activities due to the compromised immunome and risk of infecting other pathogens.

(3) A follow-up and return visit in the second and fourth weeks respectively after discharge is recommended.

CHAPTER 4

Development and Revisions of the Diagnosis and Treatment Plan of Corona Virus Disease 2019

(Tentative First to Sixth Editions)

Since December 2019, there has been an outbreak of the novel coronavirus pneumonia in Wuhan, Hubei. As the epidemic spread, such cases (officially named as COVID-19) have also been reported outside Wuhan, and cases unrelated to Wuhan have also been found. Based on the continuously in-depth understanding of the disease, National Health Commission of the People's Republic of China has released six editions of the *Diagnosis and Treatment Plan of Corona Virus Disease 2019* continuously from January 15th to February 19th, 2020, in order to further strengthen the early detection and treatment of cases, to improve the treatment ability, and to reduce hospital infection risk as much as possible at the same time. The clinical manifestations and case definitions have been refined, the diagnostic process has been optimized, and clinical management of cases is more scientific.

1 Etiology

In the initial *Diagnosis and Treatment Plan of Corona Virus Disease 2019* (Tentative First Edition), the description of coronavirus etiology was based on the understanding of physicochemical properties of previously discovered coronaviruses. With the continuously in-depth research, the second edition added *"coronaviruses cannot be effectively inactivated by chlorhexidine"*, as well asadded in the fourth edition *"2019-nCoV belongs to the genus b, with envelope, round or elliptic and often pleomorphic form, and 60–140 nm in diameter. Its genetic characteristics are obviously different from those of SARSr-CoV and MERSr-CoV.*

The homology between 2019-nCoV and bat-SL-CoVZC45 is over 85%." and "*when cultured in vitro, 2019-nCoV can be found in human respiratory epithelial cells after about 96 hours, while it takes about 6 days to isolate and culture VeroE6 and Huh-7 cell lines*", as well as "*coronaviruses are sensitive to ultraviolet rays*".

2 Epidemiological Characteristics

Based on the cases that have been searched for in the early COVID-19 spread, the descriptions of its epidemiology in the first edition were limited to that "*most cases treated currently have a exposure history of Wuhan Huanan seafood market, and some cases appear in family aggregation*".

An "*Epidemiological Characteristics*" section was added and described separately in the fourth edition. The source of infection, route of transmission and susceptible individuals were illustrated respectively: "*The major source of infection is the patients with COVID-19, and it is mainly transmitted by respiratory droplets, also via contact route. The elderly and patients with basic diseases can develop a more serious condition after infection, but there are less cases of COVID-19 in children and infants*".

Based on the fourth edition, the source of infection has been changed to that "*at present, the major source of infection is the patients with COVID-19, and asymptomatic 2019-nCoV carriers can also be the source of infection*" in the fifth edition. The descriptions of transmission routes have been changed to that "*COVID-19 is mainly transmitted by respiratory droplets and contact, and routes such as aerosol and gastrointestinal transmission remain to be confirmed*". The description of susceptible groups has also been changed to that "*Humans of all ages are generally susceptible*".

The source of infection in the sixth edition is changed from "*COVID-19 is mainly transmitted by respiratory droplets and contact*" to "*COVID-19 is mainly transmitted by respiratory droplets and close contact*", in other words, "*close*" has been added in front of "*contact*". Besides, "*Aerosol transmission is possible when humans have prolonged exposure to high concentration of aerosol in a relatively closed space*" is added in the sixth edition.

3 Clinical Characteristics

The fourth edition added *"3 to 7 days, up to 14 days"* in the description of the incubation period which has been further modified as *"1 to 14 days, and generally within 3 to 7 days"* in the fifth edition according to the results of epidemiological investigation.

The first edition described symptoms as *"fever, fatigue, dry cough, etc."* and the fourth edition added *"a few patients with symptoms such as nasal congestion, runny nose, and diarrhea"*. With the understanding of pathogenesis of critical patients, the fourth edition emphasized that severe cases were usually aggravated one week after the onset of disease, accompanying with dyspnea, and the fifth edition added hypoxemiaas a severe manifestation.

As for mild cases, the fifth edition describes them separately and changes the *"death cases more common in the elderly and those with chronic underlying diseases"*in the fourth edition tothat *"the elderly and those with chronic underlying diseases have a poor prognosis"*.

The discription of that *"the majority of patients have a good prognosis, a few patients are critically ill, and even die"* has not be changed from the first to sixth editions.

4 Laboratory Examination

That a decrease of lymphopenia is associated with severe cases has been emphasized in all editions. *"Increased troponin can be seen in some critical patients"* is gradually realized based on knowledge of *"increasing levels of liver enzyme, muscle enzyme and myoglobin, and abnormal coagulation function"*.

The fourth edition added that *"2019-nCoV nucleic acids can be detected in pharynx swabs, sputum, lower respiratory tract secretions, blood specimens"* while *"feces specimen"* where 2019-nCoV nucleic acids can also be detected is added in the fifth edition.

The sixth edition emphasizes *"To improve the positive rate of nucleic acid detection, it is recommended to collect and retain sputum in general patients except those performed with tracheal intubation (lower respiratory tract secretions should be collect); and all the specimens should be sent and tested as fast as possible."*

Chest imaging descriptions changed little from the first edition to the sixth edition.

5 Case Diagnosis

Case definitions were classified into *"observed cases"* and *"confirmed cases"* in the first edition.

The definition of observed cases is one should meet both the epidemiological exposure history (having a travel history in Wuhan, or relevant local markets, especially having direct or indirect contact history with farmers' markets two weeks before disease onset) and the clinical definition of unexplained viral pneumonia in 2007 (fever, radiographic features of pneumonia, the white blood cell count is normal or decreased in the early stage, or the lymphocyte count is decreased, or the condition is not significantly improved or progressively aggravated after 3 days of standard antibiotic treatment). For confirmed cases, the respiratory tract specimens, such as sputum and oral swab, should be collected from observed case for whole genome sequencing and it should be highly homologous with the new coronavirus.

Since increasing cases were not exposed to Wuhan Huanan seafood market and the epidemiological exposure history emphasized *"having a history of travel in Wuhan within 14 days before the disease onset"*, the second edition changed the *"observed cases"* to *"suspected cases"*, and *"having a history of travel in Wuhan within 14 days before the disease onset"* plus clinical manifestations of viral pneumonia could be considered as suspected cases. That *"the 3-day antibacterial treatment is invalid"* was deleted. The sensitivity of early detection of cases was enhanced. What's more, confirmed cases were detected by real-time fluorescence RT-PCR.

Case definitions are different between Hubei Province and other provinces except Hubei in the fifth edition. Cases are still classified into *"suspected cases"* and *"confirmed cases"* in provinces except Hubei. But *"clinically diagnosed cases"* defined as suspected cases with imaging features of COVID-19 has been added in the case classification in Hubei Province. Moreover, the criteria for suspected cases are further broadened to people with *"fever and/or respiratory symptoms"* and *"normal or decreased white blood cell count, or decreased lymphocyte count in the early stage"*.

Different case definitions for Hubei Province and other provinces except Hubei are deleted in the sixth edition and unified as *"suspected cases"* and *"confirmed cases"*.

Suspected case definitions are based on two different scenarios: (1) *"Meeting with any one of the epidemiological exposure histories and in accordance with any two of clinical manifestations (fever and/or respiratory symptoms; have the above-*

mentioned imaging features of pneumonia; the total leukocyte count was normal or decreased, or the lymphocyte count decreased in the early stage of the disease).” and (2) *“Meeting with all three of clinical manifestations (fever and/or respiratory symptoms; having the above-mentioned imaging features of pneumonia; the total leukocyte count was normal or decreased, or the lymphocyte count decreased in the early stage of the disease) but without specific epidemiological exposure history.”*.

“Severe cases” has been added to the case classification since the second edition, and the definition of critical cases remains unchanged. *“Ordinary type”* was added in the fourth edition and severe case definition was slightly modified (*“pulmonary imaging shows multiple lobar lesions, or >50% lesions progression within 48 hours and other clinical conditions requiring hospitalization”* was deleted). In the fifth edition, the definition of *“mild type”* is added, namely, the mild clinical symptoms, and no sign of pneumonia observed by imaging diagnosis.

6 Case Identification and Report

The fourth edition simplified procedures of diagnosis, reporting, identification, and referral of suspected cases.

The fifth edition separates Hubei differently with other provinces.

“For high altitude areas (above 1 kilometer), PaO_2/FiO_2 values should be adjusted based on equation of $PaO_2/FiO_2 \times$ Atmospheric Pressure (mmHg)/760” is added in *“$PaO_2/FiO_2 \leq 300$ mmHg (1 mmHg=0.133 kPa)”* in the sixth edition. Patients with *“>50% lesions progression within 24 to 48 hours in pulmonary imaging”* should be treated as severe cases.

Compared with the fourth edition, case identification and reporting procedures are same with provinces except Hubei in the fifth edition, but it emphasizes that the suspected patients should be transferred to the designated hospital as soon as possible with the permission of transfer safety. For Hubei Province, medical staff at all levels and types of medical institutions should immediately isolate and treat suspected and clinically diagnosed cases that meet the definition of the case. Every suspected or clinically diagnosed case should be isolated in a single room. And the specimens should be collected for pathogenic testing as soon as possible.

The *“Disposal requirements for clinical diagnosed case in Hubei Province”* is deleted in the sixth edition, as well as *“exclusion criteria for suspected cases”*. Standards of release of isolation for suspected cases are corresponded with *“Removal Standards of Isolation”*. *“Especially for suspected cases, rapid antigen detection, mul-*

tiple PCR nucleic acid test and other methods should be adopted to examine common respiratory pathogens" are highlighted in the sixth edition.

7 Treatment

It is suggested that *"the treatment place should be determined according to the severity of the disease"*, *"every suspected case should be treated in single room"*, and *"critical cases should be admitted to ICU as soon as possible"*.

In terms of antiviral therapy, no effective antiviral therapy is emphasized, but α-interferon aerosol inhalation, lopinavir/ritonavir, and ribavirin are recommended as trying drugs.

The fifth edition details the treatment of severe and critical cases. Respiratory support emphasizes close monitoring of finger-prick oxygen saturation, timely administration of oxygen therapy and respiratory support, especially if the condition does not improve or even worsen after *"high-flow nasal catheter oxygen therapy or non-invasive mechanical ventilation"* for a short time (1–2 hours), endotracheal intubation and invasive mechanical ventilation should be performed promptly. Blind or inappropriate use of antibiotics must be avoided, especially in combination with broad-spectrum antibiotics. It should be noted that higher doses of glucocorticoids would delay coronavirus clearance. That *"for critically ill patients with high inflammatory response, extracorporeal blood purification technology can be considered when conditions permit"* has been supplemented.

"Chloroquine phosphate (500 mg for adult, twice per day)" and *"Arbidol (200 mg for adult, three times per day)"* are added as trial drugs in the sixth edition. Combinations of ribavirin and interferon or lopinavir/ritonavir are recommended. The course of treatment with trial drugs should be ≤10 days and effects of trial drugs are recommended to be vealuated during clinical usage. Simultaneously use of three or more types of antiviral drugs is not recommended and relative drug treatment should stop if unbearable side effects occur.

As for treatment to severe and critical cases, *"convalescent plasma therapy"* is added in the sixth edition for treating rapidly developed cases, severe cases and critical cases. *"Extracorporeal blood purification technology should be considered if possible"* is changed to *"Plasma exchange, adsorption, perfusion, blood/plasma filtering and other extracorporeal blood purification technologies should be considered if possible"* for cirtical cases with severe inflammatory reactions.

8 Chinese Medicine Treatment

The third edition added traditional Chinese medicine treatment. COVID-19 also can be regarded as part of traditional Chinese medicine epidemic disease. It is caused by some epidemic pathogenic factors that located at lungs. The basic pathogenesis of COVID-19 is characterized by dampness, heat, poison, and silt. Different regions can refer to different schemes for dialectical treatment according to the disease condition, local climate characteristics, and different physical conditions. Four prescriptions and dosages were recommended, and recommendations for medical observation period, middle period and severe period were added.

9 Release of Isolation and Notes after Discharge

Standards for terminate isolation are same since the first edition to the sixth edition, which are: *"Body temperature returns to normal for more than 3 days; the respiratory symptoms recovered significantly; lung imaging shows obvious absorption and recovery of acute exudative lesion; and the detection of respiratory pathogenic nucleic acid is negative in both two consecutive tests (the sampling interval is at least 1 day)."*

The sixth edition adds *"Notes After Discharge"*:

(1) Designated hospitals should strengthen communication with basic medical institutions in patients' residence, share medical records, and forward information of discharged cases to relevant neighborhood committee and basic medical institutions.

(2) Discharged cases are recommended for continuously health monitor for 14 days, wearing facial masks, living in an ventilated single room, reducing frequency of close contact with family members, eating alone, keeping hand hygiene and avoiding outdoor activities due to the compromised immunocom and risk of infecting other pathogens.

(3) A follow-up and return visit in the second and fourth weeks respectively after discharge is recommended.

Rongmeng JIANG
Beijing Ditan Hospital, Capital Medical University, Beijing, China

PART TWO

Prevention and Control Plan of Corona Virus Disease 2019

(Source: National Health Commission (NHC) of the PRC,
Bureau of Disease Prevention and Control)

Prevention and Control Plan of Corona Virus Disease 2019

(Fourth Edition)

The 2019-nCoV belongs to the genus β coronavirus and has distinct genetic characteristics from SARSr-CoV and MERSr-CoV. Coronaviruses are sensitive to ultraviolet rays and heat, and can be effectively inactivated when environmental temperature is 56°C and lasts for 30 min, and lipid solvents such as ether, 75% ethanol, chlorine-containing disinfectant, peroxyacetic acid and chloroform except chlorhexidine. Based on current epidemiological investigations, the incubation period of COVID-19 is 1 to 14 days, and generally within 3 to 7 days. At present, the major source of infection is the COVID-19 patients, and asymptomatic 2019-nCoV carriers can also be the source of infection. The main routes of transmission are respiratory droplets and contact, while aerosol and fecal-oral transmission routes are yet to be verified. Humans of all ages are generally susceptible.

To better promote COVID-19 prevention and control work nationally, strengthen coordination of COVID-19 prevention and control institutions, complete the epidemic information monitoring and report, achieve "early detection, early report, early diagnosis, early quarantine and early treatment", decrease the spread of this epidemic, reduce morbidity and mortality, improve people's life safety and health, and maintain social stability, the fourth edition of *Prevention and Control Plan of Corona Virus Disease 2019* is updated and formulated on the basis of the third edition according to the fact that COVID-19 has been classified into the Class B communicable diseases and managed as a Class A communicable diseases, and the development of national epidemic, case epidemiology and clinical research.

1 Aims

To timely detect and report COVID-19 cases, analyze disease characteristics and exposure history, regulate the management of close contacts, provide guides to the public and specific groups for personal protection, strictly disinfect specific places, effectively prevent community spread, and reduce the adverse effect of 2019-nCoV infection on the public's health.

2 Application Scope

This plan is applicable to guiding the prevention and control work nationally and the plan will be updated based on epidemic changes and assessment results.

3 Prevention and Control Measures

3.1 Improve the Prevention and Control Mechanism, Strengthen Organizational Leadership

The prevention and control of COVID-19 should be attached with great importance. Health administrative departments at all levels should follow the administrative government and strengthen the guidance of local epidemic prevention and control work, set up expert groups for COVID-19 prevention and control. In accordance with the "prevention in the first place, integrating prevention with control, scientific guidance, timely treatment" work principle, relevant departments should be organized to formulate and improve relative work and technological solutions, and standardize the COVID-19 prevention and control work. Strengthen joint prevention and control, improve inter-communication and cooperation among departments, conduct regular consultations to analyze epidemic development and discuss prevention and control policies.

Health administrative department at all levels should be responsible for the overall guidance of epidemic control and the implementation of funds and materials.

The responsibility of CDC at all levels includes organizing, coordinating, supervising and evaluating surveillance, for collecting, analyzing, reporting and providing feedback of monitoring data; conducting training of field investigations, laboratory examinations and other professional knowledge; carrying out public health education and risk evaluation, providing personal protection methods guidelines for the public and specific people, and guiding disinfection of special places.

Medical institutions of all levels and types should be responsible for case detection, reporting, isolation, diagnosis, treatment and clinical management, as well as sample collection. Training medical staff to prevent and control nosocomial infections is also part of each institution's responsibility.

3.2 Detection and Report of Case and Public Health Emergency

All levels and types of medical institutions and disease control organizations should impose the surveillance, detection and report of COVID-19 cases and asymptomatic carriers according to the *Surveillance Plan of Corona Virus Disease 2019 Cases* (Fourth Edition) (Appendix 1).

3.2.1 Case Detection

All levels and types of medical institutions should raise awareness of the diagnosis and report of new cases during the COVID-19 surveillance and routine diagnosis and treatment. For cases with unexplained fever, cough or breathless, etc., the following information should be collected: whether the case traveled or lived in Wuhan and surrounding areas, or communities reported confirmed cases, 14 days before disease onset; whether the case has any contact with patients with fever or respiratory symptoms in areas or communities mentioned above; whether clustered onset is observed; and whether the case has contacted with any COVID-19 case.

Relevant primary organizations should organize sample test performed by professional institutions to screen high risk people who have a travel or residence history in Wuhan and surrounding areas, or other case-reported communities within the past 14 days, and have respiratory symptoms, fever, chills, fatigue, diarrhea, conjunctival congestion, etc.

3.2.2 Case Report

Detected suspected cases, clinically diagnosed cases (only in Hubei Province), confirmed cases, and asymptomatic carriers of COVID-19 should be immediately reported online by medical institutions that have established the report system, or be reported to the county (district) level CDC and send infectious disease report cards within 2 hours to other organizations without this system and local CDC is required to report the case online immediately. Medical institutions or CDCs that are responsible for direct online report should comply with the *Surveillance Plan of Corona Virus Disease 2019 Cases* (Fourth Edition)to modify case classification, clinical severity, and other information in time based on laboratory examination results and disease progress.

3.2.3 Emergency Detection and Report

Local CDC should conduct online report through the Emergency Public Reporting System (EPRS) within 2 hours once the first COVID-19 case is confirmed, or a clustered epidemic confirmed by *Surveillance Plan of Corona Virus Disease 2019 Cases* (Fourth Edition). The severity level could be "unclassified" at the beginning and later modified by health administrative department based on results of incidence investigation, risk assessment and further development.

3.3 Epidemiological Investigation

According to the *Epidemiological Investigation Plan of Corona Virus Disease 2019 Cases* (Fourth Edition) (Appendix 2), the county (district) level CDCs should complete the epidemiology investigation within 24 hours once report of suspected cases, clinically diagnosed cases (only in Hubei Province), confirmed cases, or asymptomatic carriers of 2019-nCoV by medical institutions or medical staff is received .

The county (district) level CDC should report the case questionnaire through the National Notifiable Disease Report System (NNDRS) within 2 hours, and submit the epidemiological investigation and analysis report to local health administration department and the senior CDC after completing case investigation of confirmed cases and asymptomatic carriers.

3.4 Specimen Collection and Examination

Clinical specimens of each case collected by a medical institution should be sent to a local designated laboratory, or CDC, or a third-party testing institution for pathogen test as soon as possible (see Appendix 4 for technical guidelines for laboratory examination).

Clinical specimens include patients' upper respiratory tract specimens (such as throat swabs, nasal swabs, etc.), lower respiratory tract specimens (such as respiratory tract aspirates, bronchial lavage fluid, alveolar lavage fluid, deep sputum, etc.), eye conjunctiva swabs, stool specimens, anticoagulant and serum specimens, etc. Efforts should be made to collect respiratory specimens (especially lower respiratory tract specimens) at early stage of disease onset, and serum at acute phase within 7 days of disease onset, as well as serum of recovery period at 3 to 4 weeks after disease onset.

Specimen collection, transportation, storage and test are temporarily managed as the Class B high pathogenicity pathogenic microorganisms, and should comply with the *Biosafety Management Regulation of Laboratories for Micro-organisms*, *Regulations on the Management and Transportation of Human Infectious High Pathogenicity Pathogenic Microorganism Strains or Samples (No.45, issued by the Former Ministry of Health)* and other relevant requirements.

3.5 Cases Treatment & Nosocomial Infection Prevention and Control

All cases should be treated by designated medical institutions. These institutions should ensure sufficient supply of manpower, drugs, facilities, equipment, protective appliances and so on.

Medical institutions should, in accordance with the *Technical Guidelines for Prevention and Control of 2019-nCoV Infections in Medical Institutions* (First Edition), pay attention to and strengthen the isolation, disinfection and protection work, fully implement various measures to prevent nosocomial infection, complete appointed examination and grade diagnosis procedures, and control nosocomial infection in fever clinics, emergency departments and other general wards. Suspected cases, clinically diagnosed cases (only for Hubei Province) and confirmed cases should be isolated and treated in designated hospitals with effective isolation and protective conditions. Asymptomatic infected persons should be isolated for 14 days and the isolation can be released if the nucleic acid test is negative after 7 days.

Medical institutions should strictly comply with the *Technical Standards for Disinfection in Medical Institutions* (First Edition) to clean and disinfect medical devices, polluted items, object surfaces, floors, etc., and complete air disinfection according to the requirements of *Hospital Air Purification Management Standards*. Medical wastes generated during case diagnosis and treatment should be disposed and managed in accordance with *Medical Waste Management Regulations* and *Medical Waste Management Measures of Medical and Health Institutions*.

3.6 Close Contact Tracing and Management

The county (district) level health administrative departments need to organize and implement tracing and management of close contacts with relevant departments. People who have close contact with suspected or clinically diagnosed cases (only in Hubei Province), or confirmed cases, or asymptomatic carriers, should be implemented with centralized isolation medical observations. Regions that do not meet the requirements can adopt home-based isolation medical observation. For details, please refer to *Management Plan for Close Contacts of Corona Virus Disease 2019 Cases* (Fourth Edition) (Appendix 3). Record body temperature at least twice per day and monitor whether close contacts show acute respiratory symptoms or other related symptoms and monitor disease progression. The observation period for close contacts is 14 days since the last contact with COVID-19 case or asymptomatic carriers.

3.7 Health Education and Risk Communication

The government should actively carry out public opinion monitor, popularize knowledge of epidemic prevention and control, impose mass prevention and control, timely respond to public doubts and social concerns, and make an effort to conduct epidemic prevention and control and risk communication. Strengthen health education and risk communication for specific populations, key places and large-scaled gathering activities, especially strengthen the guidance on personal protection for the public and specific groups by various methods to reduce possible contact or exposure (see Appendix 5: *Individual Protection Guidelines for Specific Populations* (Second Edition)). Health education strategies should be adjusted timely at different stages of epidemic development based on analysis of the public psychological changes and key information, and corresponding popular science propaganda should also be organized timely. Health reminder and management should be well performed when returning to school or work.

3.8 Training Healthcare Providers

Staff in medical and health institutions should be trained for COVID-19 case detection and report, epidemiological investigation, specimen collection, laboratory examination, medical treatment, nosocomial infection prevention and control, close contact management, personal protection and other contents to improve their prevention and treatment capabilities.

3.9 Improve Laboratory Examination Ability and Biological Safety Awareness

All provincial CDCs, county (district) level CDCs with laboratory examination equipment, designated medical and health institutions, and third-party test institutions should establish laboratory diagnostic methods and reserve reagents and technologies, and carry out various laboratory examinations at any time in accordance with laboratory biosafety regulations.

3.10 Timely Disinfection of Specific Places

Specific places where cases and asymptomatic infected persons have lived, such as patients' homes, isolation wards of medical institutions, transport tools and medical observation places should be disinfected timely. Assess disinfection effects of object surfaces, air and hands if necessary (see Appendix 6: *Technical Plan for Disinfection in Specific Places* (Second Edition)).

3.11 Strengthen the Prevention and Control Work of Key Places, Institutions and Populations

Strengthen the multi-departments joint prevention and control work mechanism to minimize public gathering activities, and implement measures such as ventilation, disinfection and body temperature measurement in public gathering places including stations, airports, docks, shopping malls and closed transportation vehicles such as automobiles, trains and airplanes according to local conditions.

To strengthen the COVID-19 prevention and control in collective living units, such as schools and nurseries, morning examination system and absence registration system due to illness should be established. Strengthen the prevention and control work in cities with more movable people, and prepare for prevention and control of high COVID-19 risk after the Spring Festival holiday. Health education targeted for rural farmers, students, businessmen should also be strengthened.

3.12 Scientific Classification and Community Prevention and Control Strategies

Different prevention and control strategies should be adopted by communities in different epidemic situations. Communities without any case should follow the strategy of "prevention of imported external cases", while communities with reported cases or outbreaks are suggested to comply with the strategy of "preventing cases from proliferating inwards and outputting outwards". For communities where the epidemic spreads, the strategy of "preventing the epidemic from spreading inwards and outputting outwards" should be adopted. For details, please refer to the *Prevention and Control Plan for Corona Virus Disease 2019 in Community* (Tentative Edition) in the *Notice on Strengthening Prevention and Control of Corona Virus Disease 2019 in Community* (*No.5 [2020] of the Pneumonia Mechanism*).

Appendixes

1. Surveillance Plan of Corona Virus Disease 2019 Cases (Fourth Edition)
2. Epidemiological Investigation Plan of Corona Virus Disease 2019 Cases (Fourth Edition)
3. Management Plan for Close Contacts of Corona Virus Disease 2019 Cases (Fourth Edition)
4. Technical Guidelines for Laboratory Examination of Corona Virus Disease 2019 (Fourth Edition)
5. Individual Protection Guidelines for Specific Populations (Second Edition)
6. Technical Plan for Disinfection in Specific Places (Second Edition)

Appendix 1

Surveillance Plan of Corona Virus Disease 2019 Cases
(Fourth Edition)

Cases of COVID-19 have been found in Wuhan, Hubei Province since December 2019. This Plan is formulated to give guidance on detecting and reporting cases of COVID-19 timely, ensure early detection and early reporting, and prevent epidemic spread nationally.

1　Aims

1.1 To detect and report COVID-19 cases, 2019-nCoV infected cases, and cluster outbreak cases timely;

1.2 To know the epidemic characteristics of COVID-19, and to judge and predict its developing trend in time.

2　Definition of Surveillance

2.1　Provinces except Hubei

2.1.1　Suspected Cases

The suspected cases should be diagnosed comprehensively through the combination of the following epidemiological exposure history and clinical manifestations:

(1) Epidemiology
   1) Having a history of travel or residence in Wuhan and its surrounding areas, or other communities with case reports within 14 days before the disease onset;
   2) Having a contact history with patients (a positive result of nucleic acid test of 2019-nCoV) within 14 days before the disease onset;
   3) Having a contact history with patients with fever or respiratory symptoms from Wuhan and its surrounding areas, or the communities with case reports within 14 days before the disease onset;
   4) Clustering occurrence.

(2) Clinical Manifestations
1) Fever and/or respiratory symptoms;
2) Having the imaging features of pneumonia;
3) In the early stage, a normal or decrease of total white blood cells count and a decrease of lymphocytes count can be found.

Patients who satisfy any one of the epidemiological exposure histories as well as any two of the clinical manifestations can be diagnosed as suspected cases. Patients with no definite epidemiological history can be diagnosed only if meeting the above three clinical manifestations.

2.1.2 Confirmed Cases

The suspected cases with one of the following etiological evidences can be diagnosed as confirmed cases:

(1) A positive result of the nucleic acid of 2019-nCoV by real-time fluorescence RT-PCR in respiratory tract specimens or blood specimens;
(2) The virus gene sequence of respiratory tract specimens or blood specimens is highly homologous to the known 2019-nCoV.

2.1.3 Asymptomatic Carriers

Asymptomatic carriers who present with no clinical symptom but with a positive result of the pathogens tests of 2019-nCoV in respiratory tract specimens and so on, found mainly through the investigation of cluster outbreak and tracking of source of infection.

2.1.4 Cluster Outbreak

A cluster outbreak means that more than two confirmed cases or asymptomatic carriers are found within 14 days in a small area (such as a family, a building site, a work unit, etc.), and there is a possibility of human-to-human transmission caused by close contact or by exposure to infectious source together.

2.2 Hubei Province

2.2.1 Suspected cases

The suspected cases should be diagnosed comprehensively through the combination of the following epidemiological exposure history and clinical manifestations:

(1) Epidemiology:
   1) Having a history of travel or residence in Wuhan and its surrounding areas, or other communities with case reports within 14 days before the disease onset;
   2) Having a contact history with patients (a positive result of nucleic acid test of 2019-nCoV) within 14 days before the disease onset;
   3) Having a contact history with patients with fever or respiratory symptoms from Wuhan and its surrounding areas, or the communities with case reports within 14 days before the disease onset;
   4) Clustering occurrence.

(2) Clinical Manifestations
   1) Fever and/or respiratory symptoms;
   2) In the early stage, a normal or decrease of total white blood cells count and a decrease of lymphocytes count can be found.

Regardless of epidemiological exposure histories, patients can be diagnosed as suspected cases as long as they satisfy the two clinical manifestations.

2.2.2 Clinically Diagnosed Cases
The suspected cases with imaging features of pneumonia.

2.2.3 Confirmed Cases
The clinical diagnosis cases or suspected cases with one of the following etiological evidences can be diagnosed as confirmed cases:

(1) A positive result of the nucleic acid of 2019-nCoV by real-time fluorescence RT-PCR in respiratory tract specimens or blood specimens;
(2) The virus gene sequence of respiratory tract specimens or blood specimens is highly homologous to the known 2019-nCoV.

2.2.4 Asymptomatic Carriers
Asymptomatic carriers who present with no clinical symptom but with a positive result of the pathogens tests of 2019-nCoV in respiratory tract specimens and so on, found mainly through the investigation of cluster outbreak and tracking of infectious source.

2.2.5 Cluster Outbreak

A cluster outbreak means that more than two confirmed cases or asymptomatic carriers are found within 14 days in a small area (such as a family, a building site, a work unit, etc.), and there is a possibility of human-to-human transmission caused by close contact or by exposure to infectious source together.

3 Contents

3.1 Cases Detection

(1) All types and levels of medical institutions should raise awareness of the diagnosis and reporting of COVID-19 cases during the monitoring and routine diagnosis and treatment. For cases with unexplained fever, cough or breathless, etc., the following information should be collected: whether the case traveled or lived in Wuhan and surrounding areas, or communities reported confirmed cases, within 14 days before disease onset; whether the case has any contact with patients with fever or respiratory symptoms in areas or communities mentioned above; whether clustered onset is observed; and whether the case has contacted with any COVID-19 case.

(2) Relevant primary organizations should organize sample test performed by professional institutions to screen high risk people who have a travel or residence history in Wuhan and surrounding areas, or other case-reported communities within the past 14 days, and have respiratory symptoms, fever, chills, fatigue, diarrhea, conjunctival congestion, etc.

3.2 Cases Report

Detected suspected cases, clinically diagnosed cases (only in Hubei Province), confirmed cases, and asymptomatic carriers of 2019-nCoV should be immediately reported online by medical institutions at all types and levels within 2 hours. The CDCs should investigate and verify submitted information immediately after receiving the reports, and complete the three-level confirmation review of the report information through the direct online reporting system within 2 hours. For other organizations without this system, cases should be reported to county (district) level CDCs and send infectious disease report cards out within 2 hours and local CDCs are required to report the case online immediately and correct case follow-up information.

Online report procedures are as follows: select "COVID-19" as the disease type, and select "suspected cases", "clinical diagnosis cases" (only in Hubei Province), "confirmed cases", and "positive test" in the "case classification" to report. "Clinical severity" of suspected cases, clinically diagnosed cases (only in Hubei Province), and confirmed cases should be classified as "Mild", "Ordinary", "Severe", or "Critical" according to *Diagnosis and Treatment Plan of Corona Virus Disease 2019* (Tentative Fifth Edition). A positive test refers to a person with asymptomatic infection and these cases should be selected as "asymptomatic carriers" in "clinical severity".

Reported "suspected cases" and "clinical diagnosed cases" (only in Hubei Province) should be promptly modified to "confirmed cases" or eliminated in time based on laboratory examination results. Reported "asymptomatic carriers" with clinical manifestations should be corrected in time as "confirmed case" if clinical manifestations are found. For all cases, corrections for "clinical severity" should be made in time based on disease progression and the most severe state should be regarded as final state.

3.3 Detection and Report of the Incident

Local CDC should conduct online report through the Emergency Public Reporting System (EPRS) within 2 hours once the first COVID-19 case is confirmed, or a clustered outbreak is confirmed, according to *National Emergency Plan for Public Health Emergencies* and the *National Working Standards for the Management of Related Information Reports on Public Health Emergencies* (Tentative Edition). The severity level could be "unclassified" at the beginning and is modified by health administrative department based on results of incidence investigation, risk assessment and further development, and the beginning, development, and ending of the case should also be reported online in time.

3.4 Epidemiological Investigation

The county (district) level CDC should complete the case investigation within 24 hours and conduct close contacts registration when received reports about COVID-19 suspected cases, clinical diagnosis cases (only in Hubei province), confirmed cases and asymptomatic carriers according to the *Epidemiological Investigation Plan of Corona Virus Disease 2019 Cases* (Fourth Edition) and *Management Plan for Close Contacts of Corona Virus Disease 2019 Cases* (Fourth Edition). The case investigation information of confirmed cases and asymptomatic carriers should be reported through NNDRS in time.

All county (district) level CDCs should report the epidemiological investigation and analysis report to the local health administration departments and senior CDCs in time.

3.5 Specimens Collection and Laboratory Examination

Clinical specimens of each case collected by medical institutions should be sent to local designated laboratory, or CDC, or third-party testing institution for pathogen test as soon as possible.

Clinical specimens include patients' upper respiratory tract specimens (such as throat swabs, nasal swabs, etc.), lower respiratory tract specimens (such as respiratory tract aspirates, bronchial lavage fluid, alveolar lavage fluid, deep sputum, etc.), eye conjunctiva swabs, stool specimens, anticoagulant and serum specimens, etc. Efforts should be made to collect respiratory specimens (especially lower respiratory tract specimens) at early stage of disease onset, and serum at acute phase within 7 days of disease onset, as well as serum of recovery period at 3 to 4 weeks after disease onset.

Specific requirements for clinical specimen collection and laboratory examination could be referred to the *Technical Guidance on Laboratory Testing of Corona Virus Disease 2019* (Fourth Edition).

Specimen collection, transportation, storage and test are temporarily managed as the Class B high pathogenicity pathogenic microorganisms, and should comply with the *Biosafety Management Regulation of Laboratories for Micro-organisms, Regulations on the Management and Transportation of Human Infectious High Pathogenicity Pathogenic Microorganism Strains or Samples (No.45, issued by the Former Ministry of Health)* and other relevant requirements.

3.6 Review Requirements of Laboratory Examination Results for Clustered Cases

The original specimens of more than 5 clustered cases in each region should be sent to the China CDC for review and confirmation.

Appendix 2

Epidemiological Investigation Plan of Corona Virus Disease 2019 Cases

(Fourth Edition)

This plan is formulated to better understand the epidemiological information of incidence, exposure and contact history of the COVID-19 cases, to screen close contacts, and to prevent epidemic spread.

1 Aims

1.1 To investigate the incidence and treatment, clinical characteristics, risk factors and exposure history of each case;

1.2 To identify and manage close contacts.

2 Population

COVID-19 suspected cases, clinical diagnosis cases (only in Hubei province), confirmed cases, asymptomatic carriers and cluster outbreak.

3 Contents and Methods

3.1 Case investigation

The county (district) level CDC should complete the epidemiology investigation within 24 hours since receiving relevant reports. The investigation can be carried out by consulting references, collecting related information with cases, insiders and appointed doctors. The case should be investigated first, and then the doctors, family members and insiders, if possible.

Investigation contents for suspected cases and clinically diagnosed cases (Hubei province only) are: basic information and close contacts. Only the first two parts of the questionnaire should be filled in (Box 1.1).

Investigation contents for confirmed cases and asymptomatic carriers are: basic information, disease onset and treatment, risk factors and exposure history, laboratory examinations results, close contacts, and other information showed in the questionnaire (see Box 1.1).

Judgement and management of close contacts is carried out according to the *Management Plan for Close Contacts of Corona Virus Disease 2019 Cases* (Fourth Edition).

3.2 Cluster Outbreak Investigation

Investigation should be imposed by the county (district) level CDC once cluster outbreak is confirmed according to the NNDRS and case survey results, as well as the definition in the *Surveillance Plan of Corona Virus Disease 2019 Cases*(Fourth Edition).Except for the source of infection and close contacts of all cases, the survey should also focus on investigating the epidemiological relationships among cases, analyzing the transmission chain, and filling in the basic information of the incident, beginning, development and final report in accordance with the requirements of the *National Working Standards for the Management of Related Information Reports on Public Health Emergencies* (Tentative Edition).

4 Organization and Implementation

Based on the principle of "localized management", the health administration departments at county (city, district) levels should organize disease prevention and control agencies to conduct epidemiological investigations for COVID-19 cases. An investigation team should be set up promptly, and each organization should clarify the purpose of the investigation, as well asspecify team composition and targeted responsibilities according to the investigation plan. Investigators should ensure personal safety during the investigation. The municipal, provincial and national CDCs should dispatch professionals to reach to the site as the epidemic handling needed, and conduct epidemiological investigation with the investigation team jointly.

5 Information Report and Analysis

The county (district) level CDC should report the case questionnaire or investigation results through the NNDRS within 2 hours, and submit the epidemiological investigation and analysis report to local health administration department and the senior CDC after completing case investigation for confirmed cases, or asymptomatic carriers or cluster outbreak.

Investigation Questionnaire for Corona Virus Disease 2019 Cases

(Fourth Edition)

Questionnaire No._____   ID Card No. _____

I Basic Information

The following items are same with the pandemic infectious disease report card, and the relevant information is directly transferred to case investigation information system and does not need to be re-entered. If any information is inconsistent, please check and modify it in the pandemic infectious disease report card.

1. Name: ____ ; If it's a child, the name of guardian: ____

2. Gender: ☐ Male   ☐ Female.

3. Date of birth: ____ (year/month/day), Age (if the date of birth is unknown, full age: __ years/__ months old)

4. Current address: ____ Province ____ City ____ County (District) ___Township (Street) ____ Village (Community)

5. Contact phone number: _____

6. Date of onset: _____

7. Date of diagnosis: _____

8. Type of diagnosis: ☐ Suspected case ☐ Clinically diagnosed case (Hubei Province only) ☐ Confirmed case ☐ Positive test (asymptomatic carrier)

9. Clinical severity: ☐ Asymptomatic infection ☐ Mild ☐ Normal ☐ Severe ☐ Critical

II Close Contacts

Name	Gender	Relationship With Cases	Contact Details 1	Contact Details 2	Current Address	Remarks

III Disease Onset and Treatment

10. Symptoms and signs:

☐ Fever: highest body temperature ____°C

☐ Shiver ☐ Dry cough ☐ Expectoration ☐ Stuffy nose ☐ Runny nose

☐ Sore throat ☐ Headache ☐ Fatigue ☐ Muscle soreness ☐ Joint soreness

☐ Shortness of breath ☐ Dyspnea ☐ Chest tightness ☐ Chest pain

☐ Conjunctival congestion ☐ Nausea ☐ Vomiting ☐ Diarrhea

☐ Abdominal pain ☐ Other ____

11. Complications:

☐ Yes ☐ No

If yes, please select (multiple choices): ☐ Meningitis ☐ Encephalitis ☐ Bacteremia/Sepsis ☐ Myocarditis ☐ Acute lung injury/ARDS ☐ Acute kidney injury ☐ Epilepsy ☐ Secondary bacterial pneumonia ☐ Other ____

12. Routine blood examination:

☐ No ☐ Yes

If yes, examination time: ____ (year/month/day) (if those who have examined for many times fill in the results of the first examination)

Examination result: WBC (white blood cell count) ____$\times 10^9$/L; L (lymphocyte count) ____$\times 10^9$/L; L (lymphocyte percentage) ____%; N (neutrophil percentage) ____%

13. Imaging features of pneumonia by chest X-ray examination:

☐ Unexamined ☐ No ☐ Yes

If yes, examination time: ____ (year/month/day)

14. Imaging features of pneumonia by chest CT examination :

☐ Unexamined ☐ No ☐ Yes

If yes, examination time: ____ (year/month/day)

15. Seeing a doctor after disease onset: ☐ No ☐ Yes

If yes, the date of the first visit: ____ (year/month/day), the name of the hospital: ____

16. Quarantine: ☐ No ☐ Yes

If yes, quarantine start date: ____ (year/month/day)

17. Being hospitalized:

☐ No ☐ Yes

If yes, date of admission:____ (year/month/day)

18. Accepting ICU treatment:

☐ No ☐ Yes

If yes, entry date: _____ (year/month/day)

IV Risk Factors and Exposure History

19. Whether the patient belongs to the following specific occupational groups:

    ☐ Medical staff ☐ Other staff in the hospital ☐ Pathogen microbiology testers ☐ Wild animal contact related personnel ☐ Poultry, livestock farmers ☐ Other _____

20. Whether the patient is pregnant:

    ☐ Yes ☐ No

21. Medical history (multiple choices):

    ☐ No ☐ Hypertension ☐ Diabetes

    ☐ Cardiovascular and cerebrovascular diseases ☐ Lung diseases (such as asthma, cor pulmonale, pulmonary fibrosis, silicosis, etc.) ☐ Chronic kidney disease ☐ Chronic liver disease

    ☐ Immunodeficiency diseases ☐ Other _____

    Exposure history within 14 days before disease onset or nucleic acid tests is positive:

22. Whether there is a travel or residence history of Wuhan and its surrounding areas, or other communities with case reports:

    ☐ Travel history ☐ Residence history ☐ No

23. Whether contacted with people with fever or respiratory symptoms from Wuhan and its surrounding areas, or from communities with case reports:

    ☐ Yes ☐ No

24. Whether contacted with anyone who has a history of travel or residence in Wuhan and its surrounding areas, or other communities with case reports:

    ☐ Yes ☐ No

25. Whether there is a history of contact with confirmed cases or asymptomatic carriers:

    ☐ Yes ☐ No

26. Does the patient have clustering disease in the same family, work office, nursery or school or other collective places?

    ☐ Yes ☐ No ☐ Don't know

27. Whether there is a history of medical treatment in a medical institution:

    ☐ Yes ☐ No

28. Is there any farmer's market around the place of residence (village / residential building):

☐ Yes, about____meters from home ☐ No ☐ Don't know

29. Has ever been to a farmers' market:

☐ Yes ☐ No ☐ Don't know

If yes, the case in a farmers' market is: ☐ Market employee ☐ Supplier/importer ☐ Consumer ☐ Others ____ (including food delivery, finding people, passing, etc.)

V Laboratory Examination

30. Sample collection and detection of 2019-nCoV (multiple choices):

Specimen Type	Sampling Time (year/month/day)	Test Results (positive/negative/to be tested)
Pharynx swab		
Nasal swab		
Sputum		
Tracheal secretion		
Tracheal aspiration		
Bronchoalveolar lavage fluid		
Blood		
Feces		
Others (fill in the name of the specimen)		
Not collected (do not fill in sampling time and result)		

Affiliation: _____ Investigator: _____ Date: _____

Box 1.1   Investigation Questionnaire for Corona Virus Disease 2019 Cases

Appendix 3

Management Plan for Close Contacts of Corona Virus Disease 2019 Cases

(Fourth Edition)

Based on current understanding of the 2019-nCoV infection, the incubation period for COVID-19 is up to about 14 days, and cases are transmitted from human to human, this plan is formulated to define and manage close contacts of the COVID-19 cases and effectively control the epidemic spread.

1 Criteria

Close contacts refer to people who have contacted with suspected or clinically diagnosed cases (only in Hubei Province), or confirmed cases after disease onset, or positive asymptomatic carriers, and satisfy one of the following situations, but have not taken effective protection:

1.1 Living, studying or working together, or having close contact in other situations, such as working at close range or sharing same classrooms or living in same house;

1.2 Medical staff who provide diagnosis and treatment services to patients, or family members who provide care or visit, or anyone who have similar close contact with cases, such as visiting or staying in a confined environment, or other patients and their accompanying staff in the same ward;

1.3 People who are in same transportation and have close contact with cases, including carers or accompanying persons (family members, colleagues, friends, etc.) on the same transportation, or other passengers or flight attendants who may have close contact with cases or asymptomatic carriers after investigation. See Box 1.2 for methods of defining close contacts on different vehicles.

1.4 People who are considered satisfying close contact criteria after field investigation and evaluation.

People who have been identified as close contacts are required to fill in the *Registration Form for Close Contacts of Corona Virus Disease 2019 Cases* (Table 1.1).

2 Management Requirements

2.1 Contact Management

Medical observations should be organized by health administrative departments of each region with relevant departments together. Contacts that refuse to comply should be took compulsory isolation measures by local public security organizations.

(1) The reasons, deadlines, legal basis, precautions, and disease-related knowledge of medical observations, as well as the names and contact information of institutions or medical staff that are responsible for medical observations, should be informed to close contacts in writing or orally before implementation.

(2) Centralized isolation medical observation should be adopted for close contacts, or implement home-based isolation medical observation for regions that centralized isolation is inaccessible, and pay attention to strengthen the management of home observation objects. Medical observation period is 14 days since the last unprotected contact with COVID-19 cases or asymptomatic carriers. Close contacts of confirmed cases or asymptomatic carriers should continue to be observed until the expiry even if they get negative result of the nucleic acid test during the period. Close contacts of suspected case can be released from medical observation if the suspected case is excluded.

(3) Close contacts who receive centralized or home-based isolation for medical observation should live alone and minimize contact with co-residents. Cleaning and disinfection of medical observation sites should be done to avoid cross-infection. For details, please refer to *Technical Plan for Disinfection in Specific Places* (Second Edition). People are not allowed to go out during the observation period, and should acquire permission form medical observation management staff if people have to go out, and they need to wear disposable surgical masks and avoid going to crowded places.

(4) Health risks should be notified to general contacts (e.g. living, studying or working together; taking same airplane, train or ship) other than close contacts. They should be instructed to go to hospital promptly and inform the recent history of activities if they show respiratory symptoms such as fever, cough, and diarrhea and conjunctival congestion.

2.2 Measures during Medical Observation Period

2.2.1 Following measures should be taken during medical observation period:

(1) Medical staff of designated medical and health institutions is responsible for medical observation of the close contacts of COVID-19 cases. The observation measures include: measuring body temperatures of close contacts (twice a day, in the morning and evening, respectively), inquiring about their health status, filling in the medical observation form for close contacts, filling in *Medical Observation Registration Form for Close Contacts of Corona Virus Disease 2019 Cases* (Table 1.2), and giving necessary medical help and advice. The daily summary of medical observation of close contacts can be reported based on *Daily Statistics Form of Medical Observation for Close Contacts of Corona Virus Disease 2019 Cases* (Table 1.3) and *Daily Statistics Summary Form of Medical Observation for Close Contacts of Corona Virus Disease 2019 Case* (Table 1.4).

(2) Medical staff carrying out medical observation should keep effective personal protection. Refer to *Guidance of Individual Protection in Specific Groups* (Second Edition) on protective measures.

2.2.2 During medical observation period, medical staff should immediately send the close contacts showing suspicious symptoms to designated medical institutions for clinically diagnosis and treatment, collect specimens for laboratory examinations and screening, and report to local health administrative department. The suspicious symptoms include fever, shiver, dry cough, expectoration, stuffy nose, runny nose, sore throat, headache, fatigue, muscular soreness, arthralgia, polypnea, dyspnea, chest tightness, conjunctival congestion, nausea, vomiting, diarrhea and abdominal pain. If the close contacts are diagnosed as suspected cases, clinically diagnosed cases (Hubei only) or confirmed cases, people intimately contact with them are recommended to be kept under medical observation.

2.2.3 Close contacts free of symptoms above should be removed from medical observation after the end of the period.

2.3 Centralized Medical Observation Sites

2.3.1 The requirements of the centralized medical observation sites selection and internal facilities are as follows:

(1) Centralized medical observation sites should be selected in the downwind, relatively remote, and with convenient transportation, relatively far away

from densely populated areas (in principle, greater than 500 meters), and relatively independent. Centralized quarantine should not be set up in medical institutions.

(2) The interior of the centralized medical observation site should be divided into living areas, material supply areas, and wards, etc. according to needs, and the zone mark should be clear. The site should be equipped with infrastructures to ensure people's normal life and available ventilation conditions to meet the implementation of daily disinfection measures.

(3) There should be independent septic tanks and the sewage should be disinfected before entering the municipal drainage pipe network. Pouring chlorine-containing disinfectants regularly to ensure the total residual chlorine is 10 mg/L after sterilization for 1.5 hours. The disinfected sewage should meet the *Water Pollutant Discharge Standards for Medical Institutions* (GB18466-2005). Collect the excrement in a special container and discharge it after disinfection if independent septic tanks are not available. Refer to the *General Principles of Disinfection of Epidemic Sources* (GB19193-2015) for disinfection.

2.3.2 Centralized medical observation sites should provide single rooms. Biosamples should be collected and tested in time once relative symptoms like fever, cough and other respiratory infections, diarrhea, conjunctival congestion and other symptoms appear.

Guidelines for Defining Close Contacts in Vehicles

1 Aircraft

1.1 In general, all passengers in the same row and within three rows in front and back of the case in the cabin of a civil aircraft, as well as flight attendants who provided cabin services in the above areas are close contacts. Other passengers on the same flight are general contacts.

1.2 All persons in the cabin of a civil aircraft without equipment of high-efficiency particulate filtering device.

1.3 Other persons known to have close contact with the case.

2 Train

2.1 In a fully enclosed train, all passengers and train crews from the case's compartment (hard seat/hard sleeper/soft sleeper).

2.2 In a train that is not fully enclosed, passengers who were in the same soft-bedroom as the case, or in the same hard-seat (hard sleeper) compartment and in the same area or adjacent areas with the case, and train staff who served the area.

2.3 Other persons known to have close contact with the case.

3 Car

3.1 When traveling in a fully enclosed bus, all persons in the same car as the case.

3.2 When traveling in an ordinary ventilated passenger car, passengers who sit within the three rows in front and back of the case, and drivers.

3.3 Other persons known to have close contact with the case.

4 Ship

Everyone in the same cabin with the patient and crews who served the cabin.

If the case has severe symptoms such as high fever, sneezing, coughing, and vomiting during the contact period, all persons who contacted with the case should be treated as close contacts regardless of the length of time.

Box 1.2 Guidelines for Defining Close Contacts on Different Vehicles

Table 1.1

Registration Form for Close Contacts of Corona Virus Disease 2019 Cases

Name	Contact Details	Gender	Age	Relationship with Cases	Earliest Contact Time	Last Contact Time	Contact Frequency	Contact Location	Types of Contact	Remarks (Single Exposure Time)

1. Contact frequency: i) Often ii) Usually iii) Occasionally

2. Contact location: i) Home ii) Medical institution iii) Office space iv) Entertainment place v) Others (please indicate in the form)

3. Types of contact: i) Eat together ii) Live together iii) Roommate iv) Same bed v) Staying/working together vi) Diagnosing and treating, nursing vii) Same ward viii) Entertainment ix) Others (please indicate in the form)

Table 1.2

Medical Observation Registration Form for Close Contacts of Corona Virus Disease 2019 Cases

☐ Suspected case ☐ Clinical diagnosed case ☐ Confirmed case ☐ Asymptomatic carriers

Name: _____   Contact: _____   Date of disease onset: _____

ID	Name	Gender	Age	Current Address	Date of Observation	Clinical Manifestations																										
						Body Temperature(°C)							Dry Cough							Others												
						1	2	3	4	5	6	7	1	2	3	4	5	6	7	1	2	3	4	5	6	7					

_____

_____

_____

Note:

1. This form is intended for performing medical observations of COVID-19 cases and close contacts of asymptomatic carriers.

2. In "Clinical Manifestations", fill in the measured temperature in "Body Temperature", and if "Cough" appears, click "√", otherwise click "×". Fill in the corresponding code for other manifestations: i) Chills ii) Sputum iii) Stuffy nose iv) Runny nose v) Sore throat vi) Headache vii) Fatigue viii) Muscle aches ix) Joint pains x) Shortness of breath xi) Chest tightness xii) Conjunctival congestion xiii) Nausea xiv) Vomiting xv) Diarrhea xvi) Abdominal pain

Affiliation: _____   Filler: _____   Date: _____

Table 1.3

Daily Statistics Form of Medical Observation for Close Contacts of Corona Virus Disease 2019 Cases

Street/ Community or Residence	Date of First Observation	Cumulative Number of People Observed	Medical Observation				Number of Abnormal Clinical Manifestations		Number of Cases Transformed to Confirmed Cases and Asymptomatic Carriers			Date of Last Close Contact Expected to Release Medical Observation
			Number of People Observed			Number of Released Medical Observation	Added	Accumulated	Confirmed Cases	Asymptomatic Carriers	Accumulated	
			Number	Added	Intraday	Accumulated						

Account

Note:

1. This form is applicable to medical workers for reporting medical observation of COVID-19 close contacts.

2. Abnormal clinical manifestations include: fever, cough, shortness of breath and other symptoms.

3. The cumulative numbers in the table refer to the aggregated data since the medical observations of close contacts starts.

Affiliation: _____ (Medical and Health Institutions)   Filler: _____   Date: _____

Table 1.4

Daily Statistics Summary Form of Medical Observation for Close Contacts of Corona Virus Disease 2019 Cases

Area	Date of First Observation	Cumulative Number of People Observed	Medical Observation				Number of Abnormal Clinical Manifestations		Number of Cases Transformed to Confirmed Cases and Asymptomatic Carriers			Date of Last Close Contact Expected to Released Medical Observation
			Number of People Observed		Number of Released Medical Observation							
			Number	Added	Intraday	Accumulated	Added	Accumulated	Confirmed Cases	Asymptomatic Carriers	Accumulated	

Note:

1. This form can be used for statistical summary of municipal and district CDCs.
2. Abnormal clinical manifestations include: fever, cough, shortness of breath and other symptoms.
3. The cumulative numbers in the table refer to the aggregated data since the medical observations of close contacts starts.

Affiliation: _____   Filler: _____   Date: _____

Appendix 4

Technical Guidelines for Laboratory Examination of Corona Virus Disease 2019
(Fourth Edition)

This guideline is specially developed in order to guide disease control departments at all levels and other relevant institutions to carry out laboratory examination of COVID-19 and nucleic acid detection methods that are easy to use.

1 Specimens Collection

1.1 Collection object
Suspected cases, clinically diagnosed cases (only in Hubei Province) and clustered cases of COVID-19, others who need differential diagnosis of COVID-19, or other environmental or biological materials that require further screen and test (e.g. traceability analysis).

1.2 Specimen Collection Requirements
(1) People engaged in the specimens collection of COVID-19 cases should receive biosafety training (qualified training) and possess corresponding experimental skills. Required personal protective equipment (PPE) for sampling people include: N95 or better protective masks, goggles, one-piece protective clothing, double-layer latex gloves, waterproof boots cover, and the outer latex gloves should be replaced in time if they contact with patients' blood, body fluids, secretions or excreta.
(2) The specimens of hospitalized cases should be collected by medical staff of the hospital.
(3) The specimens of close contacts should be collected by the local designated disease control and medical institutions.
(4) Multiple sampling combined with the course of the disease can be implemented according to the needs of laboratory examination.

1.3 Specimen Collection Types

Respiratory specimens (including upper and lower respiratory tract specimens) of each case must be collected during acute period; lower respiratory tract specimens (such as bronchi or alveolar lavage fluid, etc.) should be collected as a priority among severe cases; eye conjunctival swabs should be collected in cases with ocular infection symptoms; and stool specimens should be taken in cases with diarrhea symptoms. Specimens can be collected according to clinical manifestations and the interval of sampling time.

Other research materials are collected according to design requirements.

Types of specimens are as follows:

(1) Upper respiratory tract specimens include: pharynx swabs, nasal swabs, nasopharyngeal extracts and so on.

(2) Lower respiratory tract specimens include: deep cough sputum, respiratory tract extract, bronchial lavage fluid, alveolar lavage fluid, lung tissue biopsy specimens.

(3) Blood samples: try to collect 5 mL fasting blood with vacuum blood tube containing EDTA anticoagulant during acute phase of anticoagulation (within 7 days after disease onset).

(4) Serum samples: try to collect two serum samples in acute phase and convalescent stage. The first serum should be collected as soon as possible (better within 7 days since disease onset), and the second serum should be collected between the 3rd to 4th week after disease onset. A total of 5 mL serum should be collected and vacuum blood vessel without anticoagulant is suggested be used. Serum samples are mainly used for the antibody detection, which is used to confirm infectious status. Serum samples are not tested for nucleic acid.

(5) Eye conjunctival specimens: eye conjunctival wipe specimens should be collected among cases with ocular infection symptoms.

(6) Stool specimens: stool specimens should be collected among all patients with diarrhea symptoms.

1.4 Specimen Collection Methods

1.4.1 Pharynx swabs: wipe bilateral pharyngeal tonsils and posterior pharyngeal walls with two plastic rod swabs with polypropylene fiber heads at the same time. Immerse the swabs head in a tube containing 3 mL virus preservation solution (also with isotonic salt solution, tissue culture medium or phosphate buffer). Discard the tail and tighten the tube cover.

1.4.2 Nasal swabs: gently insert a plastic rod swab of polypropylene fiber head into the inner nasal and palatal region of the nasal canal, stay for a while and slowly rotate and exit. The plastic rod swab of another polypropylene fiber head is taken to collect the other nostril in the same way. The two swabs are immersed in the same tube containing 3 mL sampling solution, and the tail is discarded and the tube cover is tightened.

1.4.3 Nasopharyngeal or respiratory extracts: use a collector connected with a negative pressure pump to extract mucus from the nasopharynx or respiratory secretions from trachea. Insert the collector head into the nasal cavity or trachea, turn on the negative pressure, rotate the collector head and slowly exit, collect the extracted mucus, and rinse the collector once with 3 mL sampling solution (the collector can be replaced by connecting the child catheter with 50 mL syringe).

1.4.4 Deep cough sputum: the patient is required to cough deeply and the sputum should be collected in a 50 mL screw plastic tube containing 3 mL sampling liquid.

1.4.5 Bronchial lavage fluid: insert the collector head from the nostril or trachea socket into trachea (about 30 cm depth), inject 5 mL saline, turn on the negative pressure, rotate the collector head and slowly exit. Collect the extracted mucus and rinse the collector with sampling solution once (the child catheter can also be connected to the 50 mL syringe to replace the collector).

1.4.6 Alveolar lavage fluid: insert fiber-bronchoscope into the branch of the middle lobe of the right lung or the lingual segment of the left lung through the mouth or nose and the pharynx after local anesthesia, the top of fiber-bronchoscope is inserted into the opening of the bronchial branch, and 30–50 mL sterilized saline is added slowly per time through the trachea biopsy hole, the total amount of saline is 100–250 mL and should not exceed 300 mL.

1.4.7 Blood samples: it is suggested that 5 mL blood sample should be collected by vacuum blood tubes containing EDTA anticoagulant. Keep the sample at a room temperature for 30 minutes and centrifuge it at 1,500–2,000 rpm for 10 minutes. Plasma and blood cells are collected respectively in sterile screw plastic tubes.

1.4.8 Serum samples: 5 mL blood samples are collected by vacuum negative pressure blood collection and should be kept at a room temperature for 30 minutes, centrifuged at 1,500–2,000 rpm for 10 minutes, and collected in sterile screw plastic tubes.

1.4.9 Fecal specimens: the fecal specimens should be collected for 3–5 mL among people with diarrhea symptoms in the early stage of the disease.

1.4.10 Eye conjunctival swabs: wipe the surface of the eye conjunctiva with a swab and put the swab head into sampling tube, abandon swab tail, and suspend tube cover.

Other materials: collect according to design requirements.

1.5 Specimen Packaging

The specimens are collected and assembled in the biosafety cabinet of the Class B biosafety laboratory.

1.5.1 Specimen should be placed in a suitable-sized sample collection tube with a screw cover and a gasket and resistant to freezing. Tighten it. The sample number, type, name and sampling date should be indicated outside the container.

1.5.2 Seal the sealed specimens in a plastic bags of the suitable size and hold one specimen in each bag. The sample packing requirements should satisfy the corresponding standards of the *Technical Rules for Safe Aviation Transport of Dangerous Goods*.

1.5.3 If external specimen transportation is involved, three-layer packaging shall be carried out according to specimen type as Class A or B infectious substances.

1.6 Specimen Preservation

Samples used for virus isolation and nucleic acid test should be tested as soon as possible, and the samples that will be tested within 24 hours can be stored at 4°C; those cannot be tested within 24 hours should be stored at –70°C or below (if not available, specimens should be temporarily stored in the refrigerator at –20°C). The serum can be stored for 3 days at 4°C and longer at –20°C or lower. A special storehouse or counter should be set up to restore specimens separately. Repeated freezing and thawing should be avoided during specimen transportation.

1.7 Clinical Specimens Examination

Clinical specimens should be sent to laboratories as soon as possible after collection. Refrigerated storage methods like using dry ice are recommended if long-distance transportation is needed.

1.7.1 Clinical Specimens Submission

Clinical specimens from cluster outbreak cases of all provinces and areas should be submitted to National Institute for Viral Disease Control and Prevention of China CDC for reexamination, attached with the clinical specimen submission form (Table 1.5).

1.7.2 Pathogen and Clinical Specimen Transportation

(1) Domestic Transportation

The 2019-nCoV strains and other potentially infectious biological materials are considered as dangerous goods and classified into Class A, with a corresponding UN number of UN2814, of which packages should comply with the standard packaging requirements (PI602) of *ICAO Technical Instructions for the Safe Aviation Transport of Dangerous Goods* (Doc9284). Environmental specimens are classified into Class B, with a corresponding UN number of UN3373, of which packages should comply with the standard packaging requirements (PI650) of *ICAO Technical Instructions for the Safe Aviation Transport of Dangerous Goods* (Doc9284). Requirements for packages transported by other vehicles can refer to the above standards.

The application of transportation permit for 2019-nCoV strains or specimens should follow requirements of *Regulations on the Management and Transportation of Human Infectious High Pathogenicity Pathogenic Microorganism Strains or Samples (No.45, issued by the Former Ministry of Health)*.

(2) International Transportation

The 2019-nCoV strains and specimens transported internationally should be packaged according to the standard packaging requirements above. The application of transportation permit should follow the requirements of *Regulations for Health Inspection and Quarantine of Special Entry Exit Goods* and other relevant national and international requirements.

(3) Pathogen and Clinical Specimen Management

The 2019-nCoV strains and specimens should be managed by special-assigned personnel. Sources, types, quantity and serial numbers of the strains should be accurately recorded. Efficient measures should be taken to ensure the security of the strains and specimens and to prevent the occurrence of uselessness, malicious use, stolen, robbed, or leakage events, etc.

2 Laboratory Examination of 2019-nCoV

Conventional detection of 2019-nCoV infection is real-time fluorescence RT-PCR. All examinations for 2019-nCoV must be performed by staff with relevant technical and safe knowledges in laboratories with proper conditions. Nucleic acid detection methods in this guideline mainly target the open reading frame 1ab (ORF1ab) and nucleocapsid protein (N) of 2019-nCoV genome.

To confirm a positive case in the laboratory, the following conditions should be satisfied:

The specific real-time fluorescence RT-PCR test results are positive at both two targets of COVID-19 (ORF1ab, N) in a same specimen and resampling and retesting are required if only one positive result is observed.

2019-nCoV infection cannot be excluded by negative results, and factors that may cause false negatives should be excluded, including: poor sample quality, such as respiratory tract samples from oropharynx; too early or too late collection of samples; failure to properly store, transport and process samples; other technological problems such as virus mutation, PCR suppression, etc.

3 2019-nCoV Nucleic Acid Detected by Real-time Fluorescence RT-PCR

3.1 Aims

To standardize the working procedure of real-time fluorescent RT-PCR detection for 2019-nCoV nucleic acid, and to ensure the accuracy and reliability of the experimental results.

3.2 Application scope

Applied to real-time fluorescent RT-PCR test for 2019-nCoV nucleic acid.

3.3 Responsibility

Tester: responsible for testing samples in accordance with this test guideline.

Reviewer: responsible for reviewing whether the test operation is standard and whether the test result is accurate.

Head of the department: responsible for reviewing the department comprehensive management and test report.

3.4 Sample Reception and Preparation

Check the name, gender, age, ID and test items of the sample; any abnormal sample should be marked; samples should be stored in a −70°C refrigerator before test.

3.5 Test Items

3.5.1 Test for 2019-nCoV nucleic acid (real-time fluorescent RT-PCR)

Primers and probes targeting the ORF1ab and N gene region of 2019-nCoV are recommended.

Target one (ORF1ab):

Forward primer (F): CCCTGTGGGTTTTACACTTAA

Reverse primer (R): ACGATTGTGCATCAGCTGA

Fluorescent probe (P):5'-FAM-CCGTCTGCGGTATGTGGAAAGGTTATGG-BHQ1-3'

Target two (N):

Forward primer (F): GGGGAACTTCTCCTGCTAGAAT

Reverse primer (R): CAGACATTTTGCTCTCAAGCTG

Fluorescent probe (P): 5'-FAM-TTGCTGCTGCTTGACAGATT-TAMRA-3'

Reaction system and reaction conditions of nucleic acid extraction and real-time fluorescence RT-PCR refer to kit instructions.

3.5.2 Result Judgement

Negative: no Ct value or Ct $\geq$40.

Positive: Ct <37 could be reported to be positive.

Gray area: Ct values between 37 and 40 and retest is recommended. If the repeated Ct value <40, and the amplification curve shows obvious peaks, the sample should be judged as positive, otherwise negative.

Note: if commercial kit is used, the instructions provided by the manufacturer shall prevail.

4 Requirements for Pathogen Biosafety Experiments

According to the 2019-nCoV biological characteristics, epidemiological characteristics, clinical data and other information that are available currently, 2019-nCoV is temporarily managed as Class B pathogenic microorganisms, and the specific requirements are as follows:

4.1 Virus Cultivation

Virus cultivation refers to operations such as isolation, culture, titration, neutralization test, purification of live virus and its protein, freeze-drying of virus and recombination experiment of producing living virus. The above operations shall be conducted in the biosafety cabinet of the biosafety level 3 (BSL-3) laboratory. When extracting nucleic acid from viral culture, the addition of lysis agent or inactivating agent must be operated under protective condition and in laboratories with biosafety level equal to virus culture required. After the addition of lysis agent or inactivating agent, the viral culture can be operated referring to the protective level of uncultured infectious materials. The laboratory should apply for approval by the National Health Commission of the People's Republic of China before carrying out relevant activities.

4.2 Animal Infection Experiment

Animal infection experiment refers to the experimental operations such as infecting animals with live virus, sampling from infected animals, handling and testing infectious samples, special examination of infected animals, and disposing the excreta of infected animals. These operations should be conducted in a biosafety cabinet of the BSL-3 laboratory. The laboratory should apply for approval by the National Health Commission of the People's Republic of China before carrying out relevant activities.

4.3 Operations on Uncultured Infectious Materials

Operations on uncultured infectious materials refer to operating, such as virus antigen detection, serological detection, nucleic acid extraction, biochemical analysis, and inactivating clinical samples, on uncultured infectious materials before reliable inactivation. These operations should be conducted in the BSL-2 laboratory, and adopt personal protective condition as the BSL-3 laboratory.

4.4 Operations to Inactivate Material

Nucleic acid testing, antigen testing, serological testing, biochemical analysis and other operations of infectious materials or live viruses that are inactivated by reliable methods should be carried out in the BSL-2 laboratory. Other operations that involve inactive pathogenic viruses, such as molecular cloning, can be carried out in BSL-1 laboratory.

Table 1.5

Inspection Table for Severe Acute Respiratory Syndrome Coronavirus 2 Specimens

Affiliation of Sample Transporting (Stamp): _____   Date of Sample Transporting: _____

Deliverer: _____

Specimen ID	Specimen Types	Name	Gender	Age	Date of Onset	Date of Visiting	Date of Sampling	Specimen is/isn't from Clustered Cases§	Date of Testing	Real Time RT-PCR		Gene Sequence Homology*		Remarks
										Manufacturer	Target Gene	First-Generation	Deep Sequencing	

*"Gene Sequence Homology" is optional, and note the specific target gene sequence/whole genome sequence, and its homology with 2019-nCoV.

§Fill in YES or NO.

Appendix 5

Individual Protection Guidelines for Specific Populations
(Second Edition)

This guide is used in the prevention and control of the COVID-19 for the staff conducting epidemiological investigations, working in isolating wards and medical observation sites, and the professionals participating in transfer of cases and infected persons, cadaver handling, environmental cleaning and disinfection, specimen collection and laboratories work, etc.

1 Individual Protective Equipment and Usage

Individual protective equipment should be used by all persons who contact with or may contact with COVID-19 cases and asymptomatic carriers' contaminants (such as blood or body fluid secretions, vomit, feces, etc.) and contaminated articles or environmental surfaces, including:

1.1 Gloves
According to the work content, wear disposable rubber or nitrile gloves when entering the contaminated area or performing diagnosis and treatment operations. Disinfect in time, change gloves, and carry out hand hygiene when contacting with different patients or when gloves are broken.

1.2 Medical Protective Masks
People entering the contaminated area or performing diagnosis and treatment operations should wear medical protective masks or powered air filter respirators. Test the air tightness first when wearing the mask and ensure the medical protective mask is removed lastly when wearing multiple protective equipment.

1.3 Protective Face Screen or Goggles
Wear protective face screens or goggles if the eyes, conjunctiva and face are at risk of being contaminated by blood, body fluids, secretions, feces and aerosols when entering the contaminated areas or performing diagnosis and treatment

operations. Disinfect and dry reusable goggles in time for standby after use.

1.4 Protective Suits

Change personal clothing to overalls (surgical brush or disposable clothing, etc.) and protective clothes when entering contaminated areas or performing medical operations.

2 Hand Hygiene

Use quick-drying hand disinfectant when there is no visible contaminant, and use hand sanitizer to wash hands under water and followed by quick-drying hand sanitizer when visible contaminants are present.

Hand hygiene should be strictly complied in daily work, especially before wearing gloves and personal protective equipment, before aseptic operations, before contacting with patients' blood, body fluids and their contaminated items or contaminated environmental surfaces, and removing personal protective equipment.

3 Individual Protection of Specific Populations

3.1 Epidemiological Investigators

Wear disposable work caps, medical-surgical masks, work clothes, and disposable gloves, and keep a distance of more than 1 meter from the subject when investigating close contacts.

Wear work clothes, disposable work caps, disposable gloves, protective clothing, KN95/N95 and above particulate protective masks or medical protection face masks, protective face screens or goggles, work shoes or rubber boots, waterproof boot covers, etc., when investigating suspected cases, clinically diagnosed cases (only in Hubei Province), confirmed cases and asymptomatic carriers. Investigating these cases by telephone or video is also recommended.

3.2 Staff of Isolation Ward or Medical Observation Site

Wear work clothes, disposable work caps, disposable gloves, protective clothing, medical protective masks or powered air filter respirators, protective face screens or goggles, work shoes or rubber boots, waterproof boot covers, etc.

3.3 Workers for Transfer of Cases and Asymptomatic Carriers

Work clothes, disposable work cap, disposable gloves, protective clothing, medical protective mask or power supply filter respirator, protective face screen or goggles, work shoes or rubber boots, waterproof boot covers, etc. are recommended.

3.4 Cadaver Handlers

Work clothes, disposable work caps, disposable gloves, and long-sleeved thick rubber gloves, protective clothing, KN95/N95 or better particulate protective masks, or medical protective masks, or powered air filter respirators, protective face screens, work shoes or rubber boots, waterproof boot covers, waterproof apron or waterproof isolation clothing are recommended.

3.5 Staff for Environmental Cleaning and Disinfection

Work clothes, disposable work caps, disposable gloves, and long-sleeved thick rubber gloves, protective clothing, KN95/N95 and above particulate protective masks or medical protective masks or powered air filter respirators, protective face screens, work shoes or rubber boots, waterproof boot covers, waterproof apron, or waterproof gowns are recommended. Select a dust-toxin combination filter box or canister according to disinfectant types, and impose chemical protection such as disinfectant when using powered air-supply filter respirators.

3.6 Staff for Specimen Collection

Work clothes, disposable work caps, double gloves, protective clothing, KN95/N95 or better particulate protective masks, or medical protective masks, or powered air filter respirators, protective face screens, work shoes, or rubber boots, and waterproof boot covers are recommended. Wear a waterproof apron or waterproof gown if necessary.

3.7 Laboratory Staff

Wear at least work clothes, disposable work caps, double gloves, protective clothing, KN95/N95 or better particulate protective masks, or medical protective masks, or powered air filter respirators, protective face screens or goggles, work shoes or rubber boots, Waterproof boot cover. Wear a waterproof apron or waterproof gown if necessary.

4 Precautions for Protective Equipment Remove

(1) Try not to touch the contaminated surface when disassembling.

(2) The protective blindfold, long tube rubber shoes, and other non-disposable items taken off should be put directly into the container containing disinfectant soak; the remaining disposable items should be placed in yellow clinical waste collection bags for centralized disposal.

(3) Hand disinfection should be carried out at every step of unloading protective equipment, as well as taking off all protective equipment.

Appendix 6

Technical Plan for Disinfection in Specific Places
(Second Edition)

1 Disinfection Principles

1.1 Determination of Scope and Objects
Determine the scope, objects and time limit of on-site disinfection according to the results of epidemiological investigation. Places where confirmed cases and asymptomatic carriers have lived, such as residences, isolation wards of medical institutions and transportation tools, etc. should be disinfected at any time. All places should be implemented terminal disinfection after discharge or death of cases, or after nucleic acid test changes to negative in asymptomatic carriers.

1.2 Method Options
Medical institutions should try to choose disposable medical supplies, pressure steam sterilization should be the first choice for disinfecting non-disposable medical supplies, and non-heat resistant items can be disinfected or sterilized by chemical disinfectant or low temperature sterilization equipment. The surface of environment objects can be wiped, sprayed or soaked with chlorine-containing disinfectants, chlorine dioxide and other disinfectants. Hands and skin are suggested to be wiped by effective hand skin disinfectant or quick-drying hand disinfectant such as iodophor, chlorine-containing disinfectant and hydrogen peroxide. Indoor air can be disinfected by peroxyacetic acid, chlorine dioxide, hydrogen peroxide and other disinfectants by spraying. All disinfectant products used should meet the management requirements of the national health departments.

2 Disinfection Measures

2.1 Concurrent Disinfection
Concurrent disinfection refers to the timely disinfection of objects and places polluted by confirmed cases and asymptomatic carriers. Places where patients have lived, such as residences, isolation wards of medical institutions, medical observation places, transportation tools, etc. should be applied concurrent disin-

fection, as well as pollutants excreted by patients and relative contaminated items. Refer to terminal disinfection for sterilization methods. Spraying disinfection is not recommended in the presence of people. Places where patients are isolated can take ventilation measures (including natural ventilation and mechanical ventilation) to keep indoor air flowing. Make sure ventilate twice or three times per day for at least 30 minutes each time.

Medical institutions with sufficient conditions should place patients in the negative pressure isolation wards, isolate suspected cases in individual single rooms. Confirmed cases can be placed in the same room. Non negative pressure isolation wards should be well ventilated, and disinfect air by ventilating (including natural ventilation and mechanical ventilation) and circulating air disinfector. Air can also be disinfected by ultraviolet under unmanned conditions, the exposure time can be appropriately extended to more than 1 hour if disinfected by ultraviolet. Medical staff and accompanying staff should wash and disinfect hands after diagnosis, treatment and nursing work.

2.2 Terminal Disinfection

Terminal disinfection refers to the thorough disinfection after the source of infection leaves. Air and various items should be ensured free of pathogens after terminal disinfection. The objects of terminal disinfection include pollutants (blood, secretions, vomit, excreta, etc.) discharged from confirmed cases and asymptomatic carriers, and potentially contaminated items and places. Large area disinfection of outdoor environment (including air) is not necessary. Places where cases and asymptomatic carriers stayed for a short time without obvious pollutants do not need terminal disinfection.

2.2.1 Residence of Patient

Terminal disinfection should be performed after the patient is hospitalized or died, and a negative results of nucleic acid test of asymptomatic carriers; including floor and wall of rooms, tables, surfaces of furniture including tables and chairs, door handles, patient's tableware (drinkware), clothes, bedding and other daily necessities, toys, bathroom including toilets, etc.

2.2.2 Transportation Tools

Transportation tools should be performed terminal disinfection after cases and asymptomatic carriers leaving. Objects of disinfection include: surfaces of cabin inner wall, seats, sleepers, table and etc; tableware and drinkware; bedding and other textiles used; excreta, vomit and contaminated items and areas; toilets of trains and airplanes, etc.

2.2.3 Medical Institutions

Terminal disinfection should be completed in fever clinics and infection clinics after daily work, and isolation wards should be disinfected after the patient is hospitalized or dies, or asymptomatic carriers show negative results of nucleic acid test. Floor and walls; surfaces of tables, chairs, bedside tables, bed frames, etc.; patient's clothes, bedding and other daily necessities and related medical supplies; indoor air, etc. are suggested for terminal disinfection.

2.2.4 Terminal Disinfection Procedure

Terminal disinfection procedure complies with Appendix A of *General Principles for Disinfection of Epidemic Focus* (GB19193-2015). On-site disinfection staff should take personal protection when preparing and using chemical disinfectants.

3 Disinfection Methods for Common Contaminated Objects

3.1 Indoor Air

Terminal disinfection of indoor air in living place such as residences and isolation wards of medical institutions can refer to *Hospital Air Purification Management Code* (WS/T 368-2012). Disinfectants such as peroxyacetic acid, chlorine dioxide and hydrogen peroxide can be selected for disinfection by ultralow volume spray under unmanned conditions.

3.2 Pollutants (Blood, Secretions, Vomit, Excreta of Patients)

A small amount of pollutants can be carefully removed by dipping 5,000–10,000 mg/L of chlorine-containing disinfectant (or disinfection wipes/dry wipes that can reach high level of disinfection) with disposable absorbent materials (such as gauze, rags, etc.)

A large amount of pollutants should be completely covered with disinfectant powder or bleach powder containing water-absorbing ingredients, or fully covered with disposable water-absorbing materials and poured with a sufficient amount of 5,000–10,000 mg/L chlorine-containing disinfectant. Keep for more than 30 minutes (or use disinfection dry towel that can reach high level of disinfection), and carefully remove it. Avoid contacting with pollutants during the removal process, and the pollutants removed should be centrally disposed as medical wastes. The excreta, secretions, vomit, etc. of patients should be collected in special containers, and disinfected with 20,000 mg/L chlorine-containing disinfectant at a ratio of 1:2 in feces and medicine for 2 hours.

The surfaces of the polluted environmental objects should be disinfected after removing the pollutants. Containers containing pollutants can be soaked in disinfectant solution containing 5,000 mg/L effective chlorine for 30 minutes, and then cleaned.

3.3 Floor and Wall

Visible pollutants should be completely removed before disinfection while invisible pollutants can be wiped or sprayed with 1,000 mg/L chlorine-containing disinfectant or 500 mg/L chlorine dioxide disinfectant. Floor disinfection should be completed by spraying from outside to inside with a spray volume of 100-300 mL/m² firstly, and spraying from inside to outside again after indoor disinfection. Disinfection time should not be less than 30 minutes.

3.4 Surfaces of Objects

Visible contaminants on surfaces of treatment facilities and equipment, as well as bed fences, nightstand, furniture, doorknobs and other household items, should be completely removed before disinfection. For invisible pollutants, spraying, wiping or soaking with 1,000 mg/L chlorine-containing disinfectant or 500 mg/L chlorine dioxide disinfectant for 30 minutes are recommended.

3.5 Clothing, Bedding and Other Textiles

Aerosol generation should be avoided during item collection, and it is recommended to perform incineration as medical wastes. Items with invisible pollutants can be sterilized for reuse by circulating steam or boiling for 30 minutes, or soaking with 500 mg/L chlorine-containing disinfectant for 30 minutes and then cleaning as usual, or loading directly into the washing machine with water soluble packaging bags and washing disinfection for 30 minutes, and maintaining the effective chlorine content at 500 mg/L. The ethylene oxide can be used to disinfect expensive clothing.

3.6 Hand Hygiene

All personnel involved in field work should strengthen hand hygiene. Effective alcohol-based quick drying hand disinfectants can be used, as well as chlorine or hydrogen peroxide-based hand disinfectants under special conditions. Hand sanitizer should be used to wash hands under running water when there are visible pollutants, and then disinfect.

3.7 Skin and Mucosa

Skin contaminated by pollutants should be wiped with 0.5% iodophor or hydrogen peroxide disinfectant with a disposable absorbent material for more than 3 minutes after removing pollutants, and then cleaned with water. Mucosa should be rinsed with plenty of normal saline or 0.05% iodophor.

3.8 Tableware

After removing food residue, tableware should be boiled and sterilized for 30 minutes, or soaked in 500 mg/L chlorine-containing disinfectant with effective chlorine for 30 minutes, then be rinsed with water.

3.9 Transportation

The pollution situation should be evaluated first. Visible pollutants in trains, cars and ships should be completely removed by using disposable absorbent material with 5,000–10,000 mg/L chlorine-containing disinfectant (or can achieve high levels of disinfection wet towel/dry towel), then be sprayed or wiped with 1,000 mg/L chlorine-containing disinfectant or 500 mg/L of chlorine dioxide disinfectant disinfection for 30 minutes. When disinfecting aircraft cabins, the types and doses of disinfectants should be in accordance with the relevant provisions of Civil Aviation Administration of China (CAAC). Fabrics, cushions, pillows and sheets are recommended to be treated as clinical waste.

3.10 Household Garbage from Patients

The patients' household garbage should be treated as clinical waste.

3.11 Clinical Waste

The disposal of medical waste should comply with the requirements of the *Regulations on the Management of Medical Wastes* and the *Measures for the Management of Medical Waste in Medical and Health Institutions,* and should be handled in accordance with the conventional disposal process after packaging with double-layer yellow collection bags.

3.12 Corpse Disposal

Minimizing movement and transportation of dead patient, which should be handled timely by trained staff under strict protection. Use 3,000–5,000 mg/L chlorine-containing disinfectant or 0.5% peroxyacetic acid cotton ball or gauze to fill all open channels or wounds, such as mouth, nose, ear, anus, tracheostomy, etc. Wrap the corpse in a double layer cloth soaked with disinfectant, put it into a double layer body bag, and sent it directly to designated place by a special vehicle of the civil affairs department for cremation as soon as possible.

3.13 Matters Need Attention

Timely disinfection work should comply with the guidance of the local disease control and prevention agencies, and implemented by relevant organizations or by local disease control and prevention agencies. The concurrent disinfection and terminal disinfection of the medical institutions should be arranged by medical institutions, and the technical guidance should be provided by CDC. Non-professional personnel should receive professional training from local disease prevention and control institutions before carrying out disinfection work, take proper disinfection methods and pay attention to personal protection.

4 Evaluation of Disinfection Effect

Relevant laboratory personnel qualified for inspection and testing should evaluate disinfection effect of object surfaces, air and hands if necessary.

4.1 Surfaces

Object surfaces are sampled before and after disinfection according to *Hygienic Standard for Disinfection in Hospitals* (GB15982-2012), Appendix A, and the sampling solution after disinfection is the corresponding neutralizer.

Disinfection effect is generally evaluated based on natural bacteria, or indicate bacteria which have equal or greater resistance than existed pathogens according to actual situation. Qualified disinfection can be judged by ≥90% inactive rate of natural bacteria on the disinfection object after disinfection if taking natural bacteria as the indicator, or ≥99.9% for indicator bacteria.

4.2 Indoor Air

Air sampling are taken before and after disinfection according to the Appendix A of *Hygienic Standard for Disinfection in Hospitals* (GB15982-2012) and the sampling plate should contain corresponding neutralizer after disinfection. Disinfection can be judged as qualified if the extinction rate of natural bacteria in the air is ≥90%.

4.3 Staff's Hands

Hand sampling is taken before and after disinfection according to the Appendix A of *Hygienic Standard for Disinfection in Hospitals* (GB15982-2012), and the sampling solution after disinfection is the corresponding neutralizer. Disinfection can be judged as qualified if the inactive rate of natural bacteria on hands before and after disinfection is ≥90%.

4.4 Hospital Sewage Disinfection Effect

The evaluation is conducted in accordance with the relevant regulations of *Water Pollutant Discharge Standards for Medical Institutions* (GB18466). In areas with sustained community transmission, such as Wuhan, Hubei province, local health protection programs should be formulated for temporary special places such as centralized treatment points and centralized isolation sites.

Interpretation of the Prevention and Control Plan of Corona Virus Disease 2019

(Fourth Edition)

To better guide and promote prevention and control work of Corona Virus Disease 2019 (COVID-19) nationally, National Health Commission of the People's Republic of China revised the *Prevention and Control Plan of Corona Virus Disease 2019*, and formed the fourth edition, based on the current epidemic situation and reality. The main revisions are as follows:

1. Based on the current scientific research on the 2019-nCoV, the descriptions of the etiology section and epidemiology section of 2019-nCoV were added in the whole plan.
2. In the surveillance plan, the epidemiology description and judgment principles of suspected cases have been adjusted in the *"Definition of Surveillance"* section for provinces except Hubei. The description of that *"Wuhan or other areas where local cases continue to spread"* in the third edition has been changed to *"Wuhan and its surrounding areas or other communities with case reports"* in the fourth edition. Besides, the judgment principle of *"satisfying any one of the epidemiological histories and two of the clinical manifestations (item 1 and item 2, or item 2 and item 3)"* is adjusted to *"satisfying any one of the epidemiological exposure histories as well as any two of the clinical manifestations"*, which further increases the sensitivity of surveillance for suspected cases.
3. As for Hubei province, unique definitions of surveillance of suspected cases, clinically diagnosed cases and confirmed cases have been added, which extends range of the suspected cases in Hubei compared with other provinces.

4. In addition, the surveillance case definition is adjusted to *"confirmed cases, suspected cases and asymptomatic carriers"*, and *"mild cases"* has been deleted and included in the clinical classification. Descriptions of detecting ways, methods and relief requirements of medical observation for asymptomatic carriers have also been added in the surveillance plan.

5. What's more, the number of clustered cases has been adjusted to *"more than five"*, whose specimens need to be sent to the Chinese Center for Disease Control and Prevention for review and confirmation in the surveillance plan.

6. In the epidemiological investigation plan, the investigation contents of suspected cases are defined as basic information and the situation of close contacts, and network reports of case questionnaires are not required before the definite diagnosis, so as to reduce the work load of grassroots.

7. Management measures of close contacts and asymptomatic carriers have been adjusted. In areas where conditions are permitted, placing close contacts under intensive medical observation is required. It is emphasized that asymptomatic carriers should be placed under intensive medical observation in principle.

8. Although the route of fecal-oral transmission is still unclear, this plan has put forward corresponding measures and requirements in laboratory examinations, close contacts management, protection of specific populations and disinfection of specific sites, etc. to reduce the risk of fecal-oral transmission.

CHAPTER 3

Development and Revisions of the Prevention and Control Plan of Corona Virus Disease 2019

(First to Fourth Editions)

A number of cases with novel coronavirus pneumonia (officially named as COVID-19) have been found in Wuhan, Hubei Province since December 2019. As the outbreak spread, such cases have also been found in other parts of China and abroad. In order to guide the scientific and effective prevention and control work in each region, with the approval of the State Council, the National Health Commission of the People's Republic of China included this disease into the Class B communicable diseases and managed as a Class A communicable disease stipulated in the *Law of the People's Republic of China on the Prevention and Treatment of Infections Diseases* on January 20th, 2020, and organized China CDC and other related institutions to dynamically analyze the development of the epidemic situations and grasp the progress of prevention and control in each region. According to changes of the prevention and control situation, including the increase in clustered outbreaks in Hubei Province and Wuhan, the spread of outbreaks in provinces outside Hubei, and the detection of asymptomatic carriers, as well as the related research progress of the etiology and transmission routes of 2019-nCoV, four versions of the prevention and control plan have been revised and updated. On February 6th, 2020, the General Office of National Health Commission of the People's Republic of China issued the *Prevention and Control Plan of Corona Virus Disease 2019* (Fourth Edition) (hereinafter referred to as the *Prevention and Control Plan* (Fourth Edition)). From the First Edition to the Fourth Edition of the *Prevention and Control Plan*, the whole number of prevention and control measures has been increased from 9 to 12 and the number of appendixes has been increased from 4 to 6. The epidemiological histories and judgment principles of cases in the "Definition of Surveillance" section, the epidemiological investigation contents, as well as the judgment principles and management measures for close contacts have been major adjusted. A definition of surveillance has been added for Hubei province, and the management of possible sources of infection is more stringent. The detailed comparative analysis tables are shown (Tables 3.1–3.4).

Compared with the previous three editions, the fourth edition is revised from the perspectives of effective detecting source of infection, cutting off route of transmission and protecting susceptible individuals according to the actual work at the frontline. First, descriptions of pathogenic and epidemiological characteristics have been added in this edition for grass-roots medical personnel to better understand the transmission characteristics of 2019-nCoV, to take scientific and effective measures, and to implement prevention, control and self-protection. Second, the sensitivity of detecting the confirmed and potential source of infection is improved to a large extent. In the surveillance plan of the fourth edition, the epidemiology description and judgment principles of suspected cases have been adjusted in the *"Definition of Surveillance"* section for provinces except Hubei. The description of that *"Wuhan or other areas where local cases continue to spread"* in the third edition has been changed to *"Wuhan and its surrounding areas or other communities with case reports"* in the fourth edition. Besides, the judgment principle of *"satisfying any one of the epidemiological histories and two of the clinical manifestations (item 1 and item 2, or item 2 and item 3)"* is adjusted to *"satisfying any one of the epidemiological exposure histories as well as any two of the clinical manifestations"*, which further increases the sensitivity of surveillance for suspected cases. *"Having the imaging features of pneumonia"* is no longer a requirement for the judgement of suspected cases with epidemiological exposure history. Thus, omissive mild cases can be avoided and the possibility of detecting suspected cases can be improved in basic medical institutions. As for Hubei province, the criteria of determining suspected cases are further extended and meanwhile, a category of "clinically diagnosed cases" is added, which can improve the sensitivity of detecting suspected cases significantly. Third, the management measures of potential source of infection have been strengthened to effectively reduce the incidence of cluster cases. To reduce the spread of diseases caused by lax home quarantine, the *Prevention and Control Plan* (Fourth Edition) requires intensive isolation of close contacts and asymptomatic carriers, and home quarantine is only allowed in areas where conditions are not available. Fourth, the risk of fecal-oral transmission has been fully considered. The corresponding measures and requirements are put forward to laboratory examinations, close contacts management, specific population protection and specific sites disinfection. It is required to focus on environmental and personal hygiene, conducting excreta disinfection of the cases, conducting disinfection of medical institutions, homes, toilets and public places, and to prevent contamination of water and food by patients' stool. Fifth, the workload of case report at the grass-roots level has been reduced. The fourth edition indicated suspected cases are not required for network report on epidemiological investigation before confirmation, and raised the number requirement of clustered cases from 2 to 5, whose specimens need to be sent to the China CDC for review and confirmation.

With the in-depth understanding of 2019-nCoV and the experience accumulated in disease prevention and control, experts from the China CDC will continue to scientifically evaluate the situation of epidemic prevention and control, constantly improve the prevention and control plan, and ensure that the prevention and control work in the country is scientific, orderly, powerful and effective.

Table 3.1
Comparison of the Four Editions of Prevention and Control Plan of Corona Virus Disease 2019

Frame	Content	First Edition	Second Edition	Third Edition	Fourth Edition
Ensemble	Disease Name	Novel Coronavirus-Infected Pneumonia	Novel Coronavirus-Infected Pneumonia	Novel Coronavirus-Infected Pneumonia	Novel Coronavirus Pneumonia / Corona Virus Disease 2019
	Virus Description				Etiology and epidemiological features of new coronavirus is added.
	Route of Transmission				Although the fecal-oral transmission route has not been clarified yet, this plan has put forward corresponding measures and requirements in laboratory examination, close contacts management, specific crowd protection, and specific site disinfection, etc. to reduce the risk of fecal-oral transmission.
Aims			Add "Understanding disease characteristics and possible sources of infection".	According to the requirements of managing Class B communicable disease as Class A, it is required to "detect and report COVID-19 cases (suspected cases and confirmed cases) and infected cases (asymptomatic carriers)", and add "instruct the public and specific groups to complete personal protection, sterilize specific sites strictly, and prevent the proliferation and spread effectively".	

Continued

Frame	Content	First Edition	Second Edition	Third Edition	Fourth Edition
Prevention and Control Measures	(1) Improve the prevention and control mechanism, strengthen organizational leadership			Change the title to "Improve the prevention and control mechanism, strengthen organizational leadership". "Strengthen joint prevention and control, improve inter-communication and cooperation between each department, conduct regular consultations to analyze epidemic development and discuss prevention and control policies.", "Providing personal protection methods guidelines for the public and specific people, and guiding disinfection of special places." is added in the responsibility of CDC. The responsibility of medical institutions of all levels and types adds "Training medical staffs to prevent and control nosocomial infections".	
	(2) Detection and report of case and public health emergency	There are specific reporting methods in case report.	Delete the specific reporting methods. The relevant contents are in the "Surveillance Plan of Corona Virus Disease 2019 Cases (Fourth Edition)" (Appendix 1).	Change the title to "Case and public health emergency: detection and report"; Other changes are detailed in the surveillance plan.	A "clinically diagnosed cases" section is added for Hubei province.
	(3) Epidemiological investigation	Epidemiological investigation respondents are observational and confirmed cases of COVID-19.	Epidemiological investigation respondents are suspected cases and confirmed cases of COVID-19.	Epidemiological investigation respondents add mild cases and asymptomatic carriers of COVID-19; The investigation should complete within 24 hours while case report should be submitted within 2 hours after case investigation.	"Clinically diagnosed cases" are added as the epidemiological investigation respondents in Hubei province.

Continued

Frame	Content	First Edition	Second Edition	Third Edition	Fourth Edition
	(4) Specimen collection and examination	Clinical specimens of each case should be sent to municipal CDC for pathogen examination as soon as possible; Clinical specimens: only throat swabs are listed as the upper respiratory tract specimens.	Clinical specimens should be sent to local CDC, or medical institutions designated laboratory for pathogen examination; Type of clinical specimens: patients' upper respiratory tract specimens (such as throat swabs, nasal swabs, deep sputum, etc.); Serum specimens are added.	Pathogen examination institution adds third-party testing institution; Clinical specimens type adds eye conjunctiva swabs, stool specimens.	
Prevention and Control Measures	(5) Cases treatment & nosocomial infection prevention and control	"Multiple confirmed COVID-19 cases can be placed in the same room".	Delete "multiple confirmed COVID-19 cases can be placed in the same room".	Medical institutions should comply with the "Technical Guidelines for Prevention and Control of 2019-nCoV Infections in Medical Institutions (First Edition)", fully implement various measures to prevent nosocomial infection; Increasing the number of mild cases for isolation treatment; Emphasize mild and asymptomatic COVID-19 infections can adopt home-based isolation medical observation and treatment if a larger epidemic occurs.	Suspected cases, clinically diagnosed cases (only for Hubei Province) and confirmed cases should be isolated and treated in designated hospitals with effective isolation and protective conditions, and suspected cases, clinically diagnosed cases (only for Hubei Province) should be isolated and treated in a single room. Asymptomatic carriers should be isolated for 14 days and cannot be released until the result of nucleic acid test is negative after 7 days.

Continued

Frame	Content	First Edition	Second Edition	Third Edition	Fourth Edition
	(6) Close contact tracing and management	For people who have close contact with suspected or confirmed cases should be implemented with isolation medical observations.	For people who have close contact with confirmed cases should be implemented with home quarantine or centralized isolation for medical observations.		People who have close contact with suspected or clinically diagnosed cases (only in Hubei Province), or confirmed cases, or asymptomatic carriers, should be implemented with centralized isolation medical observations. Areas that do not meet the requirements can adopt home quarantine medical observation.
Prevention and Control Measures	(7) Health education and risk communication			Mass prevention and control is added; That "Strengthen the guidance on personal protection for the public and specific groups by various methods to reduce possible contact or exposure" is added; Descriptions of that "Health education strategies should be adjusted timely at different stages of epidemic development based on analysis of the public psychological changes and key information, and corresponding popular science propaganda should also be organized timely. Health reminder and management should be well performed when returning to school or work." are added.	
	(8) Training healthcare providers				

Continued

Frame	Content	First Edition	Second Edition	Third Edition	Fourth Edition
Prevention and Control Measures	(9) Improve laboratory examination ability and biological safety awareness	All provincial CDC, county (district) level CDC with laboratory examination equipment	*"Designated medical and health institutions"* is added.		
	(10) Timely disinfection of specific places	No such content	No such content	Add the disinfection of patients' homes, isolated wards of medical institutions, transport tools and medical observation places, and the evaluation methods of disinfection effects.	
	(11) Strengthen the prevention and control work of key places, institutions and populations	No such content	No such content	Strengthen multi-department joint prevention and control work, and implement the prevention and control work of places, institutions and populations such as stations, airports, docks, shopping malls, schools, nurseries.	
	(12) Scientific classification and community prevention and control strategies	No such content	No such content	"Different prevention and control strategies should be adopted by communities with different epidemic situations" is added.	
Appendix		4 attachments	4 attachments	6 attachments, "Guidance of Individual Protection in Specific Groups (First Edition)" and "Technical Plan for Disinfection in Specific Places (First Edition)" are added	6 attachments, "Guidance of Individual Protection in Specific Groups (Second Edition)" and "Technical Plan for Disinfection in Specific Places (Second Edition)" are added.

Table 3.2

Comparison of the Four Editions of Surveillance Plan of the Corona Virus Disease 2019 Cases

Content	First Edition	Second Edition	Third Edition	Fourth Edition
Name	Surveillance Plan of the Severe Acute Respiratory Syndrome Coronavirus 2-Infected Cases	Same as the first edition	Same as the first edition	Surveillance Plan of the Corona Virus Disease 2019 Cases
Scope	Other provinces beside Hubei and other cities in Hubei province except Wuhan. Plan for Wuhan shall separately formulate.	The monitoring work in Wuhan, Hubei province should be carried out with reference, and a specific plan should be formulated separately by the local government.	No change	All provinces
Aim	Strengthen the monitor and report of cases and clusters of infections; Understand the characteristics and development trend of the epidemic situation in China.	Timely detecting and reporting of cases and clusters of cases: Understanding the characteristics of the epidemic situation throughout the country, and timely study and determine the development trend of the epidemic situation.	No change	Timely detecting and reporting of confirmed cases, infectors and clusters.
Definition	Definition of case	Definition of case	Definition of Surveillance	Definition of Surveillance
1. Observed Cases	1. Epidemiological history: travel history in Wuhan two weeks before disease onset, or direct or indirect contact history of relevant markets in Wuhan, especially farmers' markets. 2. Clinical manifestations: (1) fever; (2) imaging features of pneumonia; (3) normal or decreased total white blood cell count or decreased lymphocyte count in the early stage of the disease; (4) no significant improvement or progressive aggravation of the disease with standard antibiotic treatment for three days. Satisfying the above two conditions	Deletion	–	–

Continued

Content	First Edition	Second Edition	Third Edition	Fourth Edition
2. Suspected Cases	–	1. Clinical manifestations: Antibacterial drugs is deleted. 2. Epidemiology: (1) Having a history of travel or residence in Wuhan within 14 days before the disease onset; (2) Having a contact history with patients with fever or respiratory symptoms from Wuhan; (3) Clustering outbreak or having epidemiological relationship with confirmed cases. 3. Definition: satisfying all three clinical manifestations as well as any one of the epidemiological exposure histories.	Epidemiology: (1) Having a history of travel or residence in Wuhan and other areas with the epidemic spread within 14 days before the disease onset; (2) Having a contact history with patients with fever or respiratory symptoms from Wuhan and other areas with epidemic spread within 14 days before the disease onset; (3) Clustering occurrence or having epidemiology connections with confirmed cases, mild cases and Asymptomatic carriers. Definition: satisfying any one of the epidemiological exposure histories as well as two clinical manifestations (item 1 and 2, or item 2 and 3), or satisfy the three clinical manifestations, regardless of epidemiological exposure histories.	1. Definition of Surveillance is divided into two parts: Hubei province and Provinces except Hubei. 2. Epidemiology is added to 4 items. (1) All areas are adjusted into Wuhan and its surrounding areas or other communities with case reports; (2) Clustering outbreak is listed as a separately item. 3. Provinces except Hubei: definition is adjusted to satisfying any one of the epidemiological exposure histories as well as any two of the clinical manifestations. 4. Hubei province: Clinical manifestations: imaging features of pneumonia is deleted; Definition: satisfy the two clinical manifestations, regardless of epidemiological exposure histories.

Content	First Edition	Second Edition	Third Edition	Fourth Edition
3. Confirmed Cases	Monitoring whether cases show respiratory symptoms or other related symptoms, and whether the gene sequence of respiratory tract specimens is highly homologous to the confirmed cases.	The suspected cases with one of the following etiological evidences can be diagnosed as confirmed cases: 1. A positive result of the nucleic acid of 2019-nCoV by real-time fluorescence RT-PCR in respiratory tract specimens or blood specimens; 2. The virus gene sequence of respiratory tract specimens or blood specimens is highly homologous to the known 2019-nCoV.	No change	Provinces except Hubei unchanged. Hubei province: Definition: the clinical diagnosis cases or suspected cases should have one of the etiological evidences.
4. Clinically Diagnosed Cases	—	—	—	Hubei province: Definition: the suspected cases should have imaging features of pneumonia.
5. Mild Cases	—	—	Definition: a positive result of the pathogens tests of 2019-nCoV in respiratory tract specimens. The clinical symptoms are mild and no pneumonia manifestation can be found in imaging.	Definition is deleted. The term is used as one of clinical classifications of clinically diagnosed cases and confirmed cases.
6. Asymptomatic Carriers	—	—	Definition: present with no clinical symptom but with a positive result of the pathogens tests of 2019-nCoV in respiratory tract specimens.	Detection method is added: by investigating cluster outbreak and tracking source of infection.

Continued

Content	First Edition	Second Edition	Third Edition	Fourth Edition
7. Cluster Outbreak	1. Suspected cluster outbreak: a confirmed case and more than one patient with fever or respiratory symptoms are found within two weeks. 2. Cluster outbreak: two confirmed cases, and there is a possibility of human-to-human transmission caused by close contact or by exposure to infectious source together.	No change	Suspected cluster outbreak is deleted. Cluster outbreak: two or more confirmed cases, mild cases or asymptomatic carriers are found within 14 days in a small area (such as a family, a work unit, etc.), and there is a possibility of human-to-human transmission caused by close contact or by exposure to infectious source together.	Definition is adjusted: two or more confirmed cases or asymptomatic carriers are found within 14 days in a small area (such as a family, a building site, a work unit, etc.), and there is a possibility of human-to-human transmission caused by close contact or by exposure to infectious source together.
Work Contents				
1. Case Detection	Without content about case detection.	Without content about case detection.	Adding Case detection methods 1. Case detection (1) Adding the sensitivity of case detection in inquiring about epidemiological history. (2) Adding the screen and sample test of high-risk people.	No change
2. Case Report	1. Report within 24 hours after confirmation. 2. The disease type is "human infected with new coronavirus", and the types of cases are "observed cases" and "laboratory-confirmed cases". 3. Notes "non-pneumonia cases". 4. The First confirmed case, suspected clustered case, and clustered case in the county should be reported as a public health emergency.	1. Report within 2 hours after diagnosis and conduct a three-level audit within 2 hours. 2. The disease type renames to "new coronavirus-infected pneumonia" and the diagnosis types are "suspected cases" and "confirmed cases". 3. Adding clinical classifications. Cases are classified according to clinical severity as "non-pneumonia cases", "mild pneumonia cases", "severe pneumonia cases" and "critical severe pneumonia cases".	1. Adding the report of mild pneumonia cases and asymptomatic carriers of COVID-19. 2. Case classification adds "positive test". 3. Cases with clinical severity of "non-pneumonia cases" change to "asymptomatic carriers". 4. Defining the most severe state of the case as its final state.	1. Adding the current address, fill in the place of residence of the case, and refine it to the detailed information of the case, such as the village, group, community, and house number. 2. Revise the clinical severity classification to "asymptomatic carriers", "mild case", "ordinary case", "severe case", and "critical case".

Continued

Content	First Edition	Second Edition	Third Edition	Fourth Edition
3. Detection and Report of the Incident	Without presented separately	Without presented separately	1. The detection and report of the incidents are listed separately from the case detection and report. 2. The First confirmed case and the clustered case of the county should be reported as a public health emergency.	No change
4. Epidemiological Investigation	Complete case investigation within 24 hours and conduct close contacts registration in time.	The case questionnaire or thematic survey report should be reported online.	No change	Report the case investigation information for confirmed cases and asymptomatic carriers online.
5. Specimen Collection and Laboratory Examination	1. Relevant pathogen tests should be done by the superior CDC with laboratory testing conditions. 2. Respiratory tract specimens (especially lower respiratory tract specimens) should be collected as soon as possible after disease onset, serum from the acute phase within 7 days and recovery period from 2 to 4 weeks after the onset of disease should also be collected.	1. The county (district) level CDC should send specimens of suspected cases to the designated CDC or medical institution for relevant pathogen tests. 2. Clinical specimen collection: adding deep sputum and anticoagulation to lower respiratory tract specimens. 3. Recovery serum was adjusted to 3 to 4 weeks after disease onset.	1. Medical institutions should collect clinical specimens of suspected or clustered cases and send to the local designated laboratory, or CDC, or third-party testing institution for pathogen test as soon as possible. 2. Eye conjunctiva swabs and stool specimens are added to clinical specimens.	Clinical specimens of suspected cases, clinically diagnosed cases (only in Hubei Province), and clustered cases should be sent for pathogen test as soon as possible.

Continued

Content	First Edition	Second Edition	Third Edition	Fourth Edition
6. Case Diagnosis Process Requirements	Case diagnosis: The first confirmed case, known as human infected with new coronavirus, in each province is subject for review by the laboratory of the China CDC and Prevention, and a provincial expert group organized by the provincial health department will make a diagnosis.	Case diagnosis process requirements: The first case of each province should be reviewed and confirmed by the China CDC or a third-party testing agency designated by the National Health Commission. The evaluation and confirmation should be carried out by the diagnosis group under the National Health Commission's Epidemic Response Disposal Leading Group.	Case diagnosis process requirements: 1. Adding that the specimens of clustered cases, the original specimens should be submitted to the provincial and national CDC for further identification. 2. Adding the content that "If there is a continuous large-scale community spread, it will be confirmed by the laboratory of the designated medical institution after being evaluated and approved by the local (municipal) level CDC".	Requirements for review of laboratory test results for clustered cases: The content is changed to that "The original specimens of 5 or more aggregated cases should be sent to the Chinese Center for Disease Control and Prevention for review and confirmation".

Table 3.3

Comparison of the Four Editions of Epidemiological Investigation Plan of Corona Virus Disease 2019 Cases

Contents	First Edition	Second Edition	Third Edition	Fourth Edition
Name	Epidemiological Investigation Plan of Novel Coronavirus-Infectious Pneumonia Cases	Same as the first edition	Same as the first edition	Epidemiological Investigation Plan of Corona Virus Disease 2019 Cases
1. Aims	1. To investigate the exposure history and possible sources of infection of the cases; 2. To identify close contacts of the cases.	1. To investigate the onset, treatment, clinical characteristics and possible sources of infection of the cases; 2. To identify and manage the close contacts of the cases.	1. To investigate the onset, treatment, clinical characteristics, risk factors and exposure history of the cases; 2. To identify and manage the close contacts.	Same as the third edition
2. Population	Observed cases, confirmed cases, clustered cases	Suspected cases, confirmed cases, clustered outbreaks	Suspected cases, confirmed cases, mild cases, asymptomatic carriers and clustered outbreaks	Suspected cases, clinically diagnosed cases (Hubei only), confirmed cases, asymptomatic carriers and clustered outbreaks
3. Contents and Methods			Add a "Clustered Outbreaks Investigation" section.	
3.1 Investigation Time Requirements	Not mentioned	Complete epidemiological investigation within 24 hours after case report.		
3.2 Possible Sources of Infection	Related exposure history of pneumonia-like patients or laboratory work	1. Delete related exposure history of pneumonia-like patients or laboratory work; 2. Add contact history of patients with fever and respiratory symptoms.	Delete this section and revise it to "Risk Factors and Exposure History".	
3.3 The Structure of the Investigation Forms	The questionnaires consist of four parts:	The forms are simplified and modified including two parts:	The questionnaires are modified into four sections:	The questionnaires are modified into five parts:

Continued

Contents	First Edition	Second Edition	Third Edition	Fourth Edition
3.3 The Structure of the Investigation Forms	1. General situation of the cases 2. The disease onset and treatment of the cases 3. Clinical manifestations, laboratory examinations, diagnosis and outcome of cases 4. Epidemiological exposure history	1. Preliminary survey information (for suspected and confirmed cases) 2. Confirmed cases survey information (for confirmed cases only)	1. Basic information 2. Disease onset and treatment 3. Risk factors and exposure history 4. Laboratory examination	1. Basic information 2. Close contacts conditions 3. Disease onset and treatment 4. Risk factors and exposure history 5. Laboratory examination
3.4 Contents of the Investigation Forms		A more detailed survey on the exposure history of farmer's market	1. Simplify and delete detailed information on farmer's market, and only keep farmer's market exposure history and wildlife contact history in the investigation forms. 2. Update epidemiological history statement: the statement of epidemiological exposure history in Question 22, 23, and 24 is revised to "Wuhan City or other areas with continuous local case transmission".	Update the epidemiological history statement again: the statement of epidemiological exposure history in Question 22, 23, and 24 is revised to "Wuhan and its surrounding areas, or from communities with case reports".
4. Organization and Implementation	Clarify the responsibilities of provincial, municipal and county-level CDCs.	Simplify and specify the investigations conducted by the local CDC.		
5. Information Report and Analysis	Case investigation forms and investigation reports are reported to the superior-level CDC step by step.	1. Case investigation forms and investigation reports should be reported online within 2 hours after the completion of investigation. 2. The specific report methods and website will be notified separately. 3. The epidemiological analysis reports should be submitted to the equative-level health administrative department and the superior-level disease control center.	After a case or outbreak investigation, the case investigation forms or investigation reports should be submitted through the online reporting system within 2 hours.	1. After a confirmed case, asymptomatic carrier or cluster outbreak investigation, the case investigation forms or investigation reports should be sent online within 2 hours. 2. It is clear that the investigation contents of suspected cases are basic information and close contact investigation, and it is no need to send the case investigation reports online before the cases are diagnosed definitely.

Table 3.4

Comparison of the Four Editions of Management Plan for Close Contacts of the Corona Virus Disease 2019 Cases

Content		First Edition	Second Edition	Third Edition	Fourth Edition
Integral Frame Structure		1 Criteria 1.1 Suspect informants 1.2 Close contacts of the cases 2 Management Requirements 2.1 Suspect informant 2.2 Close contacts of the cases	1 Criteria 1.1 Close contacts of the cases 1.2 Suspect informant 2 Management Requirements 2.1 Medical observation should be adopted for close contacts of the cases or suspect informants 2.2 Conduct health notifications for suspect informants	It is adjusted to: 1 Criteria 2 Management Requirements 2.1 Contact management 2.2 Measures during medical observation period 2.3 Centralized medical observation sites	Consistent with the third edition
Name		Management Plan for Suspected Cases and Close Contacts of the Novel Coronavirus-infected Pneumonia	Consistent with the first edition	Management Plan for Close Contacts of the Novel Coronavirus-infected Pneumonia Cases	Management Plan for Close Contacts of the Corona Virus Disease 2019 Cases
Incubation Period		"12 days"	Adjusted to "14 days"	Without revision, "14 days"	Without revision, "14 days"
Whether Human-to-human Transmission Exists		The first edition describes the cases as "no clear human-to-human transmission".	It is revised to "Human-to-human transmission exists".	Without revision	Without revision

Continued

Content	First Edition	Second Edition	Third Edition	Fourth Edition
Definition of Close Contacts	The first edition is defined as "One of the following contact situations after the onset of the case (observed and confirmed case)".	It is revised to "One of the following contact situations after the onset of the case, but without effective protection". The explanation of the contact condition has been added.	It is revised to that "one of the following contact situations occurs after the onset of illness with suspected cases, confirmed cases or mild cases, and the asymptomatic carriers show positive nucleic acid tests result, but without effective protection". Keep an explanation of exposure.	It is revised to that "Close contacts refer to people who have contacted with suspected or clinically diagnosed cases (only in Hubei Province), or confirmed cases after disease onset, or positive asymptomatic infections, and satisfy one of the following situations, but without effective protection". Compared with the third edition, added "clinically diagnosed cases (only in Hubei province)", and deleted "after the onset of mild cases". Keep an explanation of the contact.
Judgment of Suspected Exposure	The definition in the first edition is that "Persons who are exposed to processing, sales, handling, distribution, or management of new coronavirus-positive wild animals, items, and the environment without effective protection when exposed".	Consistent with the first edition	Deleted	Deleted
Determination of Close Contacts in Other Situations	People who are considered satisfying criteria after field investigation and evaluation.	It is revised to that "People who are considered eligible for contact with close contacts in other circumstances after field investigation and evaluation".	Consistent with the second edition	It is revised to that "People who are considered satisfying close contact criteria after field investigation and evaluation."
General Contacts	None	None	Add definition and treatment suggestions for general contacts.	Remain related content added in the third edition.

Continued

Content	First Edition	Second Edition	Third Edition	Fourth Edition
General Management Requirements	None	None	Add "Medical observations should be organized by health administrative departments of each region with relevant departments. Contacts who refuse to comply should be took compulsory isolation measures by local public security organizations."	Remain
Close Contact Management	Centralized isolation or home quarantine medical observation for close contacts	It is revised to "Close contacts of confirmed cases take home quarantine or centralized medical observations, and those who cannot take home quarantine medical observation can arrange centralized isolated observations".	It is revised to "Close contacts usually adopt home quarantine medical observation, and those who cannot take home quarantine medical observation can arrange centralized isolated observations."	It is revised to that "Centralized isolation medical observation should be adopted for close contacts, or home quarantine medical observation for areas that centralized isolation is inaccessible, and paying attention to strengthen the management of home observation objects."
Suspected Exposure Management	There are management contents for suspicious exposed persons, and the measures are health notification.	In addition to providing health notifications to suspicious exposed persons, management measures can also be consistent with close contacts of confirmed cases: i.e., taking home quarantine or centralized medical observations, and those who cannot take home quarantine medical observation can arrange centralized isolated observations.	Deleted	Deleted

Continued

Content	First Edition	Second Edition	Third Edition	Fourth Edition
Management Requirements for Close Contacts of Close Contact	None	None	If the close contacts are diagnosed as suspected cases, confirmed cases or mild cases, people intimately contact with them are recommended to be kept under medical observation.	It is revised to that "If the close contacts are diagnosed as suspected cases, clinically diagnosed cases (Hubei only) or confirmed cases, people intimately contact with them are recommended to be kept under medical observation."
Medical Observation Period	14 days since the last exposure or unprotected contact with COVID-19 cases	It is revised to "14 days since the last unprotected contact or suspected exposure with COVID-19 cases".	Revised content: "14 days since the last unprotected contact with COVID-19 cases or infections" Added contents: "Close contacts of confirmed cases or infections should continue to be observed until the expiry if they get negative result of the nucleic acid test during the period." "Close contacts of suspected case can be released from medical observation if the suspected case is excluded."	Revised content: "14 days since the last unprotected contact with COVID-19 cases or asymptomatic infections" Added content: none
Abnormal Clinical Manifestations During Medical Observation Period	Acute respiratory symptoms such as fever, cough, and shortness of breath. Define fever as "axillary temperature ≥ 37.3 °C"	Description of clinical manifestations is the same with the first edition. The temperature of fever is not explicitly defined in the second edition.	"Diarrhea, conjunctivitis, fatigue" and other symptoms are supplemented in abnormal clinical manifestations during medical observation period, and are consistent with clinical manifestations in Epidemiological questionnaire of the third edition. The temperature of fever is not explicitly defined in the third edition.	Consistent with the third edition

Continued

Content	First Edition	Second Edition	Third Edition	Fourth Edition
Requirements for Medical Staff During Medical Observation Period	None	None	Complemented content is that "Medical staff carrying out medical observation should keep effective personal protection. Protective measures refer to Guidance of Individual Protection in Specific Groups (First Edition)."	It is revised to that "Medical staff carrying out medical observation should keep effective personal protection. Protective measures refer to Guidance of Individual Protection in Specific Groups (Second Edition)."
Requirements for Cleaning and Disinfection of Medical Observation Sites	None	None	Complemented content is that "cleaning and disinfection of medical observation sites should be done to avoid cross-infection. For details, please refer to Technical Plan for Disinfection in Specific Places (First Edition)."	It is revised to that "cleaning and disinfection of medical observation sites should be done to avoid cross-infection. For details, please refer to Technical Plan for Disinfection in Specific Places (Second Edition)."
Centralized Medical Observation Sites	None	None	Added the requirements of the centralized medical observation sites selection and internal facilities.	The distance is revised to "farther than 500 meters in principle", other contents are consistent with the third edition.
Appendix	Three appendixes in total	Four appendixes in total, and an appendix of "Registration Form for Close Contacts of Corona Virus Disease 2019 Cases" is added.	Five appendixes in total, an appendix of "Guidelines for Defining Close Contacts on Different Vehicles" is added.	A variable of "Number of Cases Transformed to Confirmed Cases and Asymptomatic Carriers" is both added in the "Daily Statistics Form of Medical Observation for Close Contacts of Corona Virus Disease 2019 Cases" (Table 1.3) and "Daily Statistics Summary Form of Medical Observation for Close Contacts of Corona Virus Disease 2019 Cases" (Table 1.4). Others are consistent with the third edition (Box 1.1, Table 1.1, Table 1.2).

Liping WANG

Chinese Center for Disease Control and Prevention, Beijing, China

PART THREE

Guidelines for Prevention and Control of 2019-nCoV

(Source: Chinese Center for Disease Control and Prevention (China CDC))

Guidelines for Prevention and Control of 2019-nCoV

(First Edition)

Chapter Outline

- **Guide to Prevention and Control for Specific Populations I:**
  Prevention and Control Guidelines for the Elderly   118

- **Guide to Prevention and Control for Specific Populations II:**
  Prevention and Control Guidelines for Children   119

- **Guide to Prevention and Control for Specific Populations III:**
  Prevention and Control Guidelines for Students   120

- **Guide to Prevention and Control in Specific Places I:**
  Prevention and Control Guidelines for Kindergartens (or Schools)   121

- **Guide to Prevention and Control in Specific Places II:**
  Prevention and Control Guidelines for Nursing Home   122

- **Guide to Prevention and Control in Specific Places III:**
  Prevention and Control Guidelines for Work Places   123

- **Guide to Prevention and Control in Specific Places IV:**
  Prevention and Control Guidelines for Public Transports   124

- **Guide to Prevention and Control in Specific Places V:**
  Prevention and Control Guidelines for Public Places   125

- **Guide to Prevention and Control in Specific Places VI:**
  Prevention and Control Guidelines for Home Quarantine   126

- Expert Advices on Medical Management of Integrated Traditional
  Chinese and Western Medicine for Patients with Fever at Home in
  Communities (First Edition)   127

Guide to Prevention and Control for Specific Populations I:
Prevention and Control Guidelines for the Elderly

1. Ensure that the elderly acquire awareness of personal protective measures, hand hygiene requirements; avoid sharing personal items; pay attention to ventilation; and implement disinfection measures. Encourage the elderly to wash their hands frequently.

2. When the elderly have suspicious symptoms such as fever, cough, sore throat, chest tightness, dyspnea, fatigue, nausea and vomiting, diarrhea, conjunctivitis, muscle soreness, etc., the following measures should be taken:

   2.1 Self-quarantine and avoid close contact with other person.

   2.2 Health status should be assessed by medical staff and those with abnormal health conditions will be transferred to a medical institution. Wearing surgical mask is required on the way to hospital, avoiding taking public vehicles if possible.

   2.3 People who have close contact with suspicious cases should get registration immediately as well as receiving medically observation.

   2.4 Reduce unnecessary gatherings, dinner parties and other group activities, and do not arrange for centralized dining.

   2.5 If any elderly person with suspicious symptoms is diagnosed COVID-19, those who are in close contact should receive medical observation for 14 days. After the patient leaves (such as hospitalization, death, etc.), the room where he/she has lived and possible contaminated materials should be applied terminal disinfection in time. The specific disinfection procedure should be operated or instructed by professionals from local CDC, or a qualified third party. The residence without disinfection is not recommended for use.

Guide to Prevention and Control for Specific Populations II:
Prevention and Control Guidelines for Children

1. Do not go to crowded places, and do not attend parties.
2. Wear a mask when going out, and remember to remind your parents and grandparents to do so.
3. Maintain a regular schedule and healthy diet. Wash your hands carefully before meals and after defecation. Take more exercises at home with your parents.
4. Cover your mouth and nose with a paper towel or by elbow when sneezing or coughing.
5. Listen to your parents and seek immediate medical care if you have a fever or get sick.

Guide to Prevention and Control for Specific Populations III:
Prevention and Control Guidelines for Students

1. **During Winter Vacation**

    1.1 Students coming from high epidemic areas (such as Wuhan) should stay at home or in designated places for medical observation for 14 days once leaving such areas.

    1.2 All students should stay at home as instructed by schools; avoid visiting relatives and friends, attending dinner-party, and going to crowded public places, especially unventilated places.

    1.3 Students are suggested to carry out daily health monitoring and report the results to relative person according to the requirements of the community or school.

    1.4 At the end of the winter vacation, students with no suspicious symptom can return to school normally. Those with any suspicious symptom should immediately tell your school and seek medical treatment in time, and return to school after recovery.

2. **On the Way Back to School**

    2.1 Wear a medical surgical mask or a N95 mask when taking public vehicles.

    2.2 Keep hands clean all the time and reduce contact with public goods or areas in vehicles.

    2.3 Monitor health during the journey, and measure body temperature when feel feverish.

    2.4 Pay attention to health status of passengers around and avoid close contact with people who have suspicious symptoms.

    2.5 In case of having suspicious symptoms during the journey, wear a medical surgical mask or a N95 mask, avoid contacting with other people, and consult a doctor in time if necessary.

    2.6 Students who need to go to hospital during the journey should tell doctors about the travel and living history of epidemic areas, and cooperate with the doctor to carry out relevant investigations.

    2.7 Keep travel ticket information properly in case of close contact tracing.

Guide to Prevention and Control in Specific Places I:
Prevention and Control Guidelines for Kindergartens (or Schools)

1. Those who have a history of living or traveling in a high epidemic area (such as Wuhan) are suggested to have a 14 days period of home quarantine before returning to kindergartens (schools).
2. After back to kindergartens (schools), monitor the body temperature and health status every day, minimize unnecessary going-out and avoid contact with other people.
3. Wear a medical surgical mask or a N95 mask correctly when closely contacting with other teachers and students, and minimize the scope of activities.
4. Kindergartens (schools) authority should monitor the health of students closely, measuring body temperature twice a day, recording absences, early departures, and leave application. If suspicious symptoms are found among students, school authority should immediately report to the epidemic management staff and cooperate with local CDC to conduct contacts management and disinfection.
5. Schools should avoid organizing large scale gathering, strengthen ventilation and cleaning of classrooms, dormitories, libraries, activity centers, canteens, auditoriums, teachers' offices, toilets and other activity areas, where hand sanitizers and hand disinfectants should be provided.
6. School authority conducts online teaching and remedial classes for students who miss classes due to illness. For those who have delayed their exams due to illness, make-up exams should be arranged.

Guide to Prevention and Control in Specific Places II:
Prevention and Control Guidelines for Nursing Home

During the epidemic period, nursing homes are suggested to implement closed management in principle, prohibiting visitors from outsiders, keeping the residents within the nursing homes, not admitting new residents. Those who have to go out should be closely monitored after coming back.

1. Daily Preventive Measures

1.1 Ensure that the staff and the residents understand relevant knowledge, avoid sharing personal belongings, pay attention to ventilation, and perform the disinfection measures. Health records should be established for the residents and the staff, and morning check-up should be conducted every day.

1.2 Staff with suspicious symptoms should immediately go to hospital for medical examinations and not be allowed to go back to work until suspected 2019-nCoV infection and other infectious diseases have been excluded.

1.3 Establish visitor registration system, and refuse visitors with suspicious symptoms of 2019-nCoV infection. All visitors should wear surgical masks.

1.4 Keep indoor air fresh. Maintain ventilation for at least 30 minutes every half day; mechanical ventilation equipment should be equipped if opening windows is im-possible. Pay attention to avoid excessive temperature difference when opening windows in winter.

1.5 Encourage the elderly to wash hands frequently, and keep the environment clean.

1.6 Prepare isolation rooms in case of isolation treatment of the elderly with suspi-cious symptoms. Those with suspicious symptoms should be isolated in time to avoid infecting other people.

2. The Elderly with Suspicious Symptoms

The elderly with suspicious symptoms should be isolated in time in individual rooms, and his/her health status should be evaluated by medical workers. The patients should be transferred to a medical institution for treatment according to their conditions. All visiting activities should be suspended.

Guide to Prevention and Control in Specific Places III:
Prevention and Control Guidelines for Work Places

1. Staff is advised to monitor their own health and avoid going to work if he/she has suspicious symptoms of 2019-nCoV infection (including fever, cough, sore throat, chest tightness, dyspnea, fatigue, nausea and vomiting, diarrhea, conjunctivitis, muscle soreness, etc.).
2. Staff with suspicious symptoms should be required to leave work place.
3. Public goods should be cleaned and disinfected regularly.
4. Maintain air circulation in office spaces. Ensure all ventilating facilities work efficiently. Air conditioner filters should be cleaned regularly and ventilation by window opening should be strengthened.
5. Washrooms should be equipped with enough hand sanitizers and ensure the normal operation of water facilities including faucets.
6. Keep the environment clean and tidy, and clean up garbage in time.

Guide to Prevention and Control in Specific Places IV:
Prevention and Control Guidelines for Public Transports
(including aircrafts, buses, subways, trains, etc.)

1. Staff of public transports in epidemic areas should wear surgical masks or N95 masks and conduct daily health monitoring.
2. It is recommended to equip with thermometers, masks and other items in vehicles.
3. Increase the frequency of cleaning and disinfection of vehicles, and make records and signs of cleaning and disinfection.
4. Keep the vehicles well ventilated.
5. Keep the stations and the compartments clean and tidy, and clean up garbage in time.
6. Arrange rotated days off for the staff to have enough rest.

Guide to Prevention and Control in Specific Places V:
Prevention and Control Guidelines for Public Places

This guide is applicable to shopping malls, restaurants, cinemas, KTVs, internet cafes, public baths, gymnasiums, exhibition halls, railway stations, subway stations, airports, bus stops and other public places.

1. Staff in public places should monitor their own health. Do not go to work if there are suspicious symptoms of 2019-nCoV infection.
2. Staff with suspicious symptoms should be required to leave for medical care.
3. Public goods should be cleaned and disinfected regularly.
4. Maintain air circulation in office spaces. Ensure all ventilating devices work ef-ficiently. Air conditioner filters should be cleaned regularly, and ventilation by window opening should be strengthened.
5. Washrooms should be equipped with enough hand sanitizers and ensure normal operation of water facilities including faucets.
6. Keep the environment sanitary and clean, and clean up garbage in time.
7. In disease-epidemic areas, people should avoid going to public places, especially places with dense flow of people and poor ventilation.

Guide to Prevention and Control in Specific Places VI:
Prevention and Control Guidelines for Home Quarantine

1. **Living Space Arrangement**
   1.1 People with suspicious symptoms need to live in well-ventilated single rooms and refuse all visits.
   1.2 Family members should live in different rooms. Stay at least one meter away and sleep in separate beds if conditions do not permit. People with suspicious symptoms should avoid activities, limit living space, and ensure the shared space (such as kitchens and bathrooms) is well ventilated (keeping windows open).

2. **Caregiver Arrangements**
   It is best to have a regular family member who is healthy and free of chronic diseases to take care of patients.

3. **Spreading Prevention**
   Family members live with people who have suspicious symptoms should wear medical surgical masks that closely fit the face. Keep hands clean at all times and avoid direct contact with body secretions, and do not share any items that may cause indirect contact infection.

4. **Treatment of Contaminants**
   Used gloves, paper towels, masks, and other wastes should be placed in a special garbage bag in patient's room and marked as contaminants before discarded.

5. **People with any of the following symptoms should immediately stop home quarantine and seek medical treatment in time.**
   5.1 Breathing difficulties (including increasing chest tightness, suffo-cation and breathless after activities).
   5.2 Disorders of consciousness (including lethargy, nonsense, inability to distin-guish between day and night).
   5.3 Diarrhea.
   5.4 Fever with a body temperature higher than 39°C.
   5.5 Other family members develop suspected symptoms of 2019-nCoV infection.

Expert Advices on Medical Management of Integrated Traditional Chinese and Western Medicine for Patients with Fever at Home in Communities (First Edition)

Corona virus disease 2019 (COVID-19) epidemic was detected in Wuhan City, Hubei Province in December 2019. Current data shows that most patients are ordinary cases. At the same time, the late winter and early spring each year is also the period of high incidence of cold and flu. Thus, recently, there are a high number of crowds in fever clinics and wards. Some fever patients chose home isolation due to fear of cross-infection risk. According to the *Diagnosis and Treatment Plan of Corona Virus Disease 2019* (Tentative Fourth Edition), *Prevention and Control Plan of Corona Virus Disease 2019* (Third Edition) and *Scheme for Diagnosis and Treatment of Influenza (2019)*, etc., we make this recommendation to guide patients with fever under home quarantine.

1. Screening Recommendations of Home Quarantine for Patients with Fever

Respiratory infections have high incidence in the winter and spring. Typical cold, flu, and COVID-19 can cause fever, but the symptoms are different. For example, the typical cold usually manifests as obvious upper respiratory tract symptoms such as sneezing, runny nose and throat discomfort, but systemic symptoms are mild, such as no fever or only transient fever. The flu usually causes high fever, severe systemic symptoms, with chills, headache, systemic aches, nasal congestion, runny nose, dry cough, chest pain, nausea and loss of appetite. The COVID-19 manifests as fever, fatigue, and dry cough. A small number of patients have symptoms such as nasal congestion, runny nose, and diarrhea.

If fever, cough and other symptoms occur, people are suggested to be placed under home quarantine once the following conditions are met:

1.1 Mild symptoms, with body temperature <38°C; with no obvious shortness of breath, chest tightness, difficult breathing; and with stable vital signs such as breathing, blood pressure, and heart rate.

1.2 Without severe basic diseases of respiratory and cardiovascular systems and severe obesity.

2. Medical Management Recommendations for Patients with Fever at Home

2.1 More rest, keep balanced diet without fat, oil and sugar.

2.2 Drink warm water rather than cold beverage to ensure normal spleen and stomach function.

2.3 Avoid overuse or inappropriate use of antimicrobials.

2.4 Wear masks correctly, have meals separately from family members, and keep a distance of more than 1.5 meters from family members.

2.5 People with chills can choose Chinese patent medicines with antipyretic and cold-dispelling properties.

2.6 People with chills, fever, muscle soreness, and cough can choose Chinese patent medicines with heat clearing and detoxifying, ventilating the lung and arresting cough.

2.7 People with fatigue, nausea, decreased appetite, and diarrhea can choose Chinese patent medicines of dehumidification.

2.8 People who have fever with obvious sore throat can choose Chinese patent medicines with clearing heat and detoxifying.

2.9 Fever with constipation can additionally use diarrhea-inducing, fever-appeasing preparations.

2.10 When a body temperature is higher than 38.5°C, physical cooling measures such as warm towels or ice sticks can be taken. People with this condition are recommended to take antipyretic and analgesics or take antipyretic and detoxifying medicines.

The specific drugs above can refer to the recommended drugs in the *Diagnosis and Treatment Plan of Corona Virus Disease 2019* (Tentative Fourth Edition).

3. Family Prevention and Control Measures for Patients with Fever

3.1 Recommend a period of 7 days for home quarantine.

3.2 Keep the indoor environment clean and ventilated for half an hour, one to three times per day. Pay attention to keep warm when ventilating.

3.3 Wear masks correctly, cover mouth with tissues or elbow rather than hands when coughing and sneezing, wash hands frequently (do not touch mouth, nose, eyes, etc. with dirty hands) and put down the toilet lid before flushing.

3.4 Avoid gatherings, dine-parties and reduce stay time in crowded places as shorter as possible.

3.5 People with fever, cough and other symptoms should be aware of the methods of self-quarantine, such as single-room isolation; if not permitted, patients should keep a distance of at least 1.5 meters from family members;

close the door to avoid air convection between rooms; do not use central air conditioner.

3.6 On the way to hospital, all people should wear masks.

3.7 Masks used by patients should be sealed in a bag and then placed in a trash can.

4. Main Symptoms Monitoring of Patients with Fever during Home Quarantine

4.1 Measure and record body temperature at least twice a day.

4.2 Whether there is chest tightness, shortness of breath, polypnea, increased heart rate and so on.

4.3 Whether the digestive system symptoms such as diarrhea and vomiting are aggravated.

5. Suggestions on the Management of Abnormal Symptoms When during Home Quarantine

5.1 If the following conditions occur, it is recommended to go to the designated hospitals and fever clinics to seek medical care:

(1) High body temperature lasts for more than 2 hours.

(2) Chest tightness and shortness of breath occur.

5.2 If respiratory frequency ≥30 breaths/min occurs, accompanied with respiratory difficulty and cyanosis of the lips, etc., immediately dial 120 for help. Patient should be transferred to the designated hospital or fever clinic by emergency medical staff.

This Expert Advice will be further revised based on evidence from clinical practice and should be used specially according to the relevant characteristics of each region.

Interpretation of the Guidelines for Prevention and Control of 2019-nCoV

(First Edition)

Since December 2019, increasing cases of corona virus disease 2019 (COVID-19) have gradually been diagnosed in Wuhan, Hubei Province. With the spread of the epidemic, infected cases have also been reported in other regions of China and abroad. On January 8th, 2020, the pathogen of this outbreak was identified as the novel coronavirus 2019. On February 1st, 2020, National Health Commission of the People's Republic of China issued the *Guidelines for Prevention and Control of 2019-nCoV* (First Edition) (hereinafter referred to as the *Prevention and Control Guidelines*), of which main contents are interpreted as follows.

Contents of prevention and control guidelines in specific populations and specific places, and experts' advice on medical management of integrated traditional Chinese and Western medicine for patients with fever at home are included in the First Edition of *Prevention and Control Guidelines*.

1 The Guidelines Focus Prevention and Control Suggestions on the Elderly, Children and Students.

1.1 In China, there are a large number of aged people, who are the high-risk susceptible population of infectious diseases due to their weakening immune functions. Similarly, the elderly account for the most of critical cases in this epidemic. The elderly should understand personal protective knowledges, wear masks correctly, wash hands frequently, strengthen ventilation and disinfection of residences, and avoid gatherings during the epidemic. People who have a fever or close contact with suspicious cases should get registration in the community or local medical institutions timely, and receive quarantine and active health monitoring. After the confirmed cases leave, their residences should be thoroughly disinfected by the local CDC or a qualified third party.

1.2 Children are also the susceptible individuals, should avoid going to crowded places, wear masks when going out, wash hands when coming back. In addition, children should maintain a healthy diet and seek medical care timely when feeling sick.

1.3 Students who have a history of living or traveling in high epidemic areas should stay at home or in designated places for 14 days quarantine. During the winter vacation, students should stay at home, reduce times of gathering, carry out daily health monitoring and report the results according to the local requirements. After returning to school, those with any suspicious symptom should initiatively report it to school and then seek medical treatment in time. On the way back to school, students should always wear medical masks, avoid contacting with other people. Those with suspected symptoms should initiatively tell the truth about the travel and residence history, and cooperate with corresponding personnel to perform investigations when seeking medical care. Students are required to keep the travel ticket information to help relevant sectors to conduct possible close contact investigations.

2 The Guidelines Propose Suggestions on Kindergartens (or Schools), Nursing Home, Office Space, Vehicles, Public Places and Home Quarantine.

2.1 Kindergartens (or Schools) belong to a kind of children and adolescents densely populated places. Students who have a history of living or traveling in a high epidemic area or have suspected symptoms are suggested to have a 14-day period of home quarantine before returning to school. School authorities should monitor students' body temperature twice a day and require students to wear masks correctly. If suspicious symptoms are found among students, school offices should cooperate with medical and health institutions to conduct management and disinfection for the close contacts. Large collective activities or gathering should be cancelled and ventilation and cleaning of relevant places should be strengthened.

2.2 Nursing institutions are suggested to implement a closed management of no going out, no visiting and no admitting for new residents. Ventilation and warmth of the rooms as well as publicity and education of prevention and control knowledge and health monitoring for the elderly and staff should be reinforced. Staff with suspicious symptoms should immediately go to hospital for medical examinations and are not allowed to go back to work until the suspected 2019-nCoV infection and other infectious diseases have been excluded. Isolation rooms for future treatment of the elderly with suspicious symptoms should be prepared. Those with suspicious symptoms should be isolated in time and transferred to medical institutions for treatment in accordance with relevant regulations. At the same time, all visiting activities should be suspended.

2.3 In office space and public places (shopping malls, restaurants, cinemas, KTV, internet cafes, public baths, gymnasiums, exhibition halls, railway stations, subway stations, airports, bus stops, etc.), health monitoring of staff should be reinforced, and those with suspicious symptoms are not allowed to work. Disinfection of public goods and ventilation of public places should be conducted regularly. Keep the environment sanitary and clean, and clean up the garbage in time. Ensure enough hand sanitizer in the washrooms and normal operation of water facilities. During the epidemic, people should avoid going to public places, especially to densely populated places of poor ventilation.

2.4 Staff of vehicles (including aircraft, buses, subways, trains, etc.) should wear masks, and keep rotated days off. In the vehicles, thermometers and masks should be provided, ventilation and tidy and clean should be maintained, garbage should be cleaned up timely, and the frequency of cleaning and disinfection should be increased.

2.5 People with suspicious symptoms need to live in a single room during home quarantine or isolation. If conditions do not permit, they should stay at least one meter away from family members. All members should wear marks, wash hands frequently, and ensure the shared space well ventilated. Goods used by the members with suspected symptoms should be dropped in a special garbage bag and marked as a contaminant. People or their family members with symptoms like dyspnea, consciousness change, diarrhea and fever $\geq$39°C should seek immediate medical treatment.

3 The Guidelines Propose Expert Advice on Medical Management of Integrated Traditional Chinese and Western Medicine for Patients with Fever at Home.

3.1 Respiratory infections have high incidence in winter and spring. Thus, patients without basic diseases or severe obesity are suggested to be placed under home quarantine if they have mild symptoms including mild fever and cough, body temperature <38°C, and stable vital signs.

3.2 During home quarantine, patients should take a good rest, have a balanced and light diet, drink warm water frequently, and suit the remedies to different situations (fear of cold, nausea or pharyngalgia) according to the recommendations in the *Diagnosis and Treatment Plan of Corona Virus Disease 2019*.

3.3 Patients should monitor body temperature at least twice a day. Once the conditions, such as high body temperature lasting for more than 2 hours, chest tightness, shortness of breath, respiratory frequency ≥30 times/min and dyspnea occur, patients should immediately go to or dial 120 and seek help to be transferred to the designated hospital for medical treatment.

3.4 Protective measures for family members and garbage disposal of quarantined personnel should also be well implemented.

Peng WANG

Chinese Preventive Medicine Association, Beijing, China